The Balanced Approach To Total Wellness

By

Taya Day

Table of Contents

Introduction...9

A Nation of Dieters

The Perfect Storm of Weight Gain and Poor Health

Say Goodbye to Fad Diets

Your Attitude Matters Most

Chapter 1: Goal Setting...30

A Life-Changing Shift is Waiting to Happen

Whatever it Takes to Get You Going

Small Steps Make a Huge Difference!

Nobody Likes To Do Chore

Making Tough Choices

Looking Beyond the "Fat" Problem

It's More Expensive to Be Overweight

Thinking Beyond the Weight Loss

Another Big Fat Excuse We Tell Ourselves

Diets are temporary

Focusing on the wrong thing

Fat and unhealthy is the easiest thing to be in North America.

Our Relationship With Food Matters

Triggers for Food

A Complete Holistic Path of Health & Fitness

Goals Often Arise from Deep within Us

The Secret Why Most Diets Don't Work

Diets Create an Even Larger Problem Later

Why People Fail at Real Weight Loss

The Balanced Approach To Total Wellness

Why People Succeed with Their Health Goals

Assessing Where You Are Now

My Initial Assessment of Those I Train & Work With

Creating Your Vision

Instituting The Law of Attraction with Weight Loss

More Brainstorming & The Law of Attraction

Coming up with a Realistic plan for YOU

Tracking Your Progress

Holding yourself Accountable (Creating Measurable Benchmarks)

Helpful Recommendations

Creating a Sustainable Mindset for the Long Haul

Consider Five Easy Things You Can Do Today to Support Natural Weight Loss

Your Winning Mind Set & Motivation

Find Good Reasons to Stay Motivated

Time to Take a Different Approach

How to Support your Will Power

Provide Incentives For Your Success

Take a look Around: Your Environment

Who We Socialize with is Important

Buy In from Those Around You

Your Lifestyle Matters

Why do we eat when we are stressed?

Stress Factors that Impact our Health & Fitness

Life changing stress factors which are prominent:

Ways to Tackle Stress

Sleep & Hunger – A New Perspective

Finally, what are benefits of being fit and healthy?

Chapter 2: Nutrition..130

The Importance of Nutrition

How to Shop For Food

Consider the following when it comes to our purchasing habits:

Making Bad Choices Difficult to Make

Balancing Protein, Carbs, & Fats

Our Water Intake

Sports Drinks and Beverages

Eating Good Fats

Coffee/Caffeine

Why You Should Switch to a Healthy Non-Caffeinated Alternative

The Dairy Problem

Other Factors Regarding Milk

Detoxing Your Body

How do "detox and cleanse" programs work?

Do Detox Regimens Generate Weight Loss?

How to Stop Sugar Addiction

Hormones and Our Health

The Portions We Eat Always Needs to Be a Consideration For Us

Fats

Restaurant Eating

Some Strategies When You Eat Out

Age Factors

A Life Long Goal of Health

What if I break my health routine?

Integrating your Nutrition and Diet with Your Exercise

The Basics of a Gluten-Free Diet and How it Can Help Us

More on Gluten Labeling

Watch for cross-contamination

Risks of Gluten Free Food Consumption

Not getting enough vitamins

Not sticking to the gluten-free diet

The Gluten Conclusion

Eliminate All Processed Foods

Organic and Genetically Modified Food

Read the Labels

Buying Organic Is Essential But Shop Smart

What about "Natural" label products?

Behavioral Relationship with Food

You knew it was coming: A few Do's and Don'ts

Eating Organic is essential

Learning from your Personal assessment

Chapter 3: Fat Loss/Diet.......................................**198**

Be Smart, Avoid the Fat Trap

Don't Count Calories

Remember, Stick to Portion Sizes

Carbs - Reducing Body Fat

Good & Bad Carbs

Avoid White Sugar or Fructose

Taya's Fat Loss Tips

Supplements - Reducing Body Fat

Avoiding Common Pit Falls

Whey Protein

Chapter 4: Diets...217

Athlete Diet Example Diet

Paleo Diet Example 2

Meatless (Lacto-ovo Diet)

Meal Planning & Choices

Before we begin a meal plan:

Some Tips on Food Planning:

Are you too busy to prepare meals?

Chapter 5: Fitness...227

Idea of Problem Spots (belly, love handles, thighs, flabby back

Intensity Workouts:

Longer Fat Burning Workouts

Strength Training/Workouts

Fine Tuning Your Fitness Routine

Burning Fat Tips

Cooling Down & Warm Ups

The Workouts

Top Training tips for Body Composition

More on your metabolic rate

Soon you your body will adapt to these positive changes.

Allow Some Time for Your Body to Rest

Chapter 6 - Lifestyle/Personal Care Products.......246

Effects of Stress on Health

Herbal Remedies

Supplements To Promote Better Sleep

Physical-Mental Activities:

The Beauty Product Lie

Choose Your "Natural" Cosmetics Carefully.

Real Dangers of SLS—Rumors Aside

Links Between SLS, Ethylene Oxide, 1,4 Dioxane, and Cancer

Clean up and green up your daily cleansing and moisturizing regimen.

How can you get your skin clean by washing it with ingredients like that?

How to Evaluate Your Toxicity

Women & Men Versus Chemical Toxicity

Final Tips and Tricks to Lighten Your Toxic Load

BPA Plastic Bottles

Personal Care and Cleaning Products, Brands (Whole Foods, Noah's, Online)

Chapter 7: Hormones...**268**

Hormonal Imbalance

How Hormones Effect Your Weight

A Loss of Sleep

How to Maintain Healthy Hormonal Balance

Hormones and Proper Diet, and the Impact on our Health

Hormone Beneficial Foods

Supplements that support our hormones

Conclusion..**279**

About Taya Day..**282**

References...**283**

Disclaimer: The essential purpose of this book is to educate and it is bought and sold with the understanding that the author, publisher, and vendors shall not be liable or responsible for any injury caused or alleged to be caused directly or indirectly by the information contain in this book. The nutrition, diet, and exercise programs are not to be substituted from personalized advice and recommendations from your health practitioner. Before any exercise and diet program it is strongly recommended that you consult your personal physician, especially if you are pregnant or nursing, or are elderly, or have a chronic physical or medical condition. As with any program, if you feel dizzy or ill, or have any physical discomfort, you should stop immediately and consult with your doctor.

Introduction

Congratulations! If you have picked up this book then you have taken the first and most powerful small step towards improving your fitness, body composition, state of mind and the overall quality of your health!

As a fitness trainer, I have seen many lives transformed, bodies healed, and confidences improved, by people who were *willing* to make just small, but essential life- changing steps towards the life they wanted.

Many people who I have come across have decided to simply move a few degrees in a different and positive direction, consistently over time, often result in the creation of a new, healthier, and happier life.

The good news is that it doesn't matter where you are with regards to your fitness – whether you are just starting out or whether you are in very good shape. There is always room to continue to do our best.

You are probably no stranger modern day life as I know it. Today, more than ever, we find ourselves over-stressed, over-worked, and over-burdened with life's demands. These demands can put a tremendous amount of pressure our system – our mind, our body, and soul.

In addition this extreme pressure constantly applied can accelerate aging and chip away at our physical abilities, mental clarity, emotional well-being, and overall health.

Overtime, all these negatives compounded upon one another can make us feel depressed, tired, and hopeless. Unfortunately, too many people live and function in a dark fog brought on by stress, depression, ill health, and negative feelings with regards to our body image – for years!

The battle of our health and fitness always moves into our head, where the real war is either lost or won. And yet, the good news is that our bodies nearly always respond to the healthy things we do. Whether it's a short walk, a healthy meal, or time in meditation, our body sends signals down to each of our cells that it's time for them to wake up and get moving.

We have trillions of cells in our body. Every last one of them is designed to do a specific thing to maintain our health. When our cells are running on all cylinders and feeling good, our mind is in calm and focused, and our spirit is in a much happier place, we begin to realize just how wonderful we can feel. Our body responds in kind. The truth is that we always perform our best when our body, mind, and soul are optimally working in sync with each other. And that wonderful feeling brought on by good health and fitness is where we were meant to thrive.

Wherever we happen to be in our lives today, we can make simple daily improvements to make us healthier and happier, resulting in feeling and looking better today and tomorrow. In this book, I will discuss a number of different things that we can do get us where we want to be – starting today!

The Topics in this book will include:

- **Vision & Goal Setting**
- **Creating a new Attitude & New Mind Set**
- **Focusing on Optimal Nutrition**
- **Fine Tuning Your Fitness Routine**
- **Steps To Burning Your Fat**
- **Provide you with Several Sample Diet Plans that work**
- **Discuss Diet and Product Substitutions that are Available to You**

None of these things happen in any particular order because frankly, they all happen at once. Starting off with a great goal and positive attitude is certainly essential in the beginning, but if it isn't sustained *throughout* the process, then you will burnout quickly and be unable to reach your goals.

In addition, maintaining a fitness routine while eating healthy is essential too. All these elements are simply spokes in a wheel that will help us move forward in reaching our goals. None of them is less important than the next.

This book is not simply about diet and exercise.
Rather this book is about *radically* changing and developing a lifestyle that promotes a healthy mind, body, and spirit. I promise you that if you are willing to walk with me on this journey, you will have the potential to see many wonderful improvements in a very short time.

This book is also about success – your success. It is about your new success story waiting to happen. If you stick with me, I have a confident feeling that we will succeed together in this journey to total health, fitness, and wellness.

Therefore, let's take a moment to understand the course we will be taking. This book is organized in the following way:

First, we will first discuss and review the importance of our attitude and vision, and how making small but necessary adjustments, as well as making the lifestyle changes that you need to be successful in weight loss, feeling better, and looking great, will all lead to realizing our goals.

To do this, you have to believe that you can achieve better health by the actions that you take. In other words, if you can believe it and take well thought out action steps, then you can do lose the weight you want and feel better about your health too! If you don't believe you can do it – or if you doubt yourself, then you will make it that much more challenging.

This book is about taking back your health and putting the control back in your hands. If you are sitting in the "average" person's chair, you might not imagine that you have control to change your life. After all, how many diets have you tried over the course of your adult life? How many times have you tried to get back into shape? Do I need to ask how many times you have failed to achieve your goals? The fact is that we often fail despite all our efforts because the diets and programs were never intended to be successful in the long run!

This book will help you break the diet-weight gain cycle so that you can actually achieve the weight and fitness goals that have been illusive to so many of you.

A Nation of Dieters

Nearly 50 percent of people are actively trying to lose weight in the United States at any given time! This is incredible when you think about it because that means that hundreds of millions of people in U.S. and Canada are on a diet – a diet that will usually fail. It's a sad but true story. Unfortunately, for all the effort, nearly 70% of people gain the weight back – and more! (1)

There is nothing else to call it but a tragedy of epic proportions! No doubt, a well-calculated tragedy that nets billions of dollars in profits by people up and down the supply chain – from agricultural food giants, corn-syrup producers, chemical producers, fast food chains, marketers, to diet plan specialists, surgical doctors who implant bands, etc. The list goes on and on. Everyone is making money off a horrible epidemic and health emergency.

It is an emergency with no end in sight. Did you know that the average American woman spends nearly 35 years of her life dieting? For the average American man it is nearly 30 years. Imagine 30 to 35 years to life - of struggling, of diets that deny us pleasure, increase our guilt, empty our wallets, and provide nothing but shattered dreams and an unbalanced body in its wake? It's true. A majority of us are living this collective nightmare of being unable to move forward in our health, fitness and the inability to lose weight. (2)

But why? After all, we all want to lose weight and be healthy, right?

I like to follow the money. There is big money in getting people to become overweight (high sugar snack foods, fast food, additives that may induce hunger are added to our favorite meals, etc., to name just a few). And there is even more in the following decades of trying to get them back "normal" with fad diets, fad meals, restrictive diets, diet pills, etc. None of it has worked. I would imagine that you have probably struggled too in this arena since you are reading this book. Collectively, we are gaining weight faster than in any other time period in our recorded history. Our clothes are getting bigger, our homes are getting bigger, our chairs are getting bigger, and our health expenses are certainly getting bigger!

The Perfect Storm of Weight Gain and Poor Health

When we consider all of the factors that contribute negatively to our health and fitness: stress, chemical and pollution exposure, genetically modified foods, refined sugar, hormone additives, lack of sleep, lack of exercise, confusing labeling, and in increasingly sedentary lifestyle, we have entered into the "perform storm" of ill health.

There are certain factors beyond caloric intake and beyond the math that we will explore here in this book. However, to bluntly tell you – many of us have unfortunately lost before we even set out to accomplish our health goals. The cards aren't simply stacked in our favor. Did you know that if you were to speak to your child one-on-one, reminding your child of the importance of healthy eating at every meal between the ages of 3 years old and 18, you would still be outgunned by tens of thousands of messages to eat other sugary snacks that significantly contribute to our obesity problem?

The fact is that we are inundated with images, jammed with images that we are constantly not good enough, don't look pretty enough, not "man" enough, not "lady" enough, and that you especially don't deserve a healthy great looking body unless you buy their products!

Well, I am here to tell you that *you are good enough*, you are beautiful enough, and you are special enough to deserve the very best. When people begin to believe that lie that they have been subtly and explicitly told in a variety of different messages every day, our attitudes are affected, our goals are cut down, our feelings of empowerment shrivels, and we then desperately look for other things to make us feel better – like watching television, eating fatty foods, and drinking alcoholic and sugary drinks, to name a few.

Say Goodbye to Fad Diets

If you're like the rest of us, then over the years you have probably tried many, many different diets, programs, fads, and gizmos to lose weight and tackle your fitness. You've also probably tried many different foods to help you to achieve your dieting goals: bland crackers, tasteless bars, and liquid diets. And for whatever reason, they have all seemed to fail or fall short, right?

Well, I am going to ask you to try one more time - to believe *one more time* that you can do it and hope that you can achieve significant fitness improvements in your life. You may have failed many times before, but it's never too late to start again! Let me say this again: **It's never too late to try and lose the weight you want again!**

The point is that you have to keep trying and you have to keep believing that you can make a difference in your own life, and in your own health! There are so many things we struggle for – our mortgage, keeping up with the bills, being there for our children and family. This time, I am going to ask you one more time – to invest in yourself. You can do it – and I will walk you through it.

If you get nothing else from this book except this very point: that fad diets don't work and they actually cause you to gain the weight even more weight, then it will be worth the price of this book alone! Do it now – say "goodbye" to fad diets forever! They don't work!

Your Attitude Matters Most

What if I told you that you that the key to losing the weight you want, gaining the muscle mass you want, living a more successful life is right in your very front pocket? You probably would snicker or laugh at me, right?

Well, it may not be in your pocket, but it's certainly in a convenient place that you have the power to possess. All you have to do is simply reach for it.

The key to your success is your attitude. Your attitude has the enormous potential to unlock and open doors in your life and in those around you.

Without sounding too cliché, consider all the achievements and accomplishments you have reached in your own life. If you really stop to think about all the great things that you have personally accomplished – all of the triumphs you have achieved, you will see this more clearly: Your perseverance and your passion for those things that you have accomplished stemmed from your attitude. Am I right? How could you achieve all the important victories in your life without a positive attitude? I don't think it can be done.

And here is the secret: To do meaningful things in our life, we have to let go of the un-meaningful. Sounds simple, right? It is actually a lot hard than it sounds.

We have to acknowledge that our attitude and perspective play a big role in our ability to achieve our dreams. Just like anything else, you need to have the right attitude to push us through the valleys - the times where we want to give up, where we think that the journey is too long and where there is seemingly very little hope left to change your path.

You have got to believe that you can create a new body and a jump to a new level of better health for yourself! Your attitude, like a tiller on a boat, will help guide you in the direction you want to go in.

Certainly every one of us is different, every person has a particular body type, and will experience different results, but the truth is that an attitude pointed in the right direction with action taken can lead to drastic improvements. Even small shifts in attitude about the food we eat, our shopping routine, our exercise regimen, and our levels of stress, can have a significant impact over time.

I know that weight loss or working on your body might be difficult because you may have tried and failed before. I have been there with you. That's why in this book, **I am not proposing a new "fad" diet**, because who really needs another fad diet? Rather, I am proposing a lifestyle shift that leads to vastly radical results over time.

Let me just say this again: Your ultimate success in losing weight, in changing your physique, improving your health numbers, are essentially based on your attitude. Not just any attitude, but the right attitude that is positive, focused, and determined to improve. Like a spark, you have to focus on nurturing that attitude, protecting it from getting blown away, or stamped out. An attitude that keeps you moving forward even if you have a "bad day" or a couple bad days in a row is more important than anything anyone can ever do for you.

Ultimately, your attitude starts and stops with you. You can have every fitness expert and trainer in the world at your disposal, but if your attitude isn't where it should be to facilitate the change you want, then it will all be futile.

Your attitude is ultimately the "mortar" or the glue that holds your habits together. Your habits, in turn, are building blocks to your general lifestyle. And it's your lifestyle that that we will operate within - to ultimately change your health, your look, and ultimately the way you feel in inside about yourself.

This process doesn't happen overnight. It never does! The sugary-sweet fantasy that diets today emphasize is this fact: That you can lose enormous amounts of weight while maintaining your lifestyle. If we stop to think about this for a second: Do we seriously think we can lose 30 lbs. of weight eating potato chips and watching television every night?

Everyone struggles to maintain a healthy lifestyle, healthy habits, and healthy attitudes. We are constantly bombarded with images that are unhealthy, constantly being over-fed, over-medicated, over-stressed, and over-worked. Oftentimes, the easiest thing to seemingly do is order that greasy pizza, basket of fries, or devour that bucket of ice-cream. We often find ourselves lacking options and choices due to our personal circumstances. But we can make some changes today, tomorrow, and the next day. Small changes that can tip things back in our favor.

These all add up. And they will eventually create the change we are looking for in our lives.

You see our body is ready to respond to the healthy choices we make. It is ready to jump on a break in the fat intake, the sugar intake – to flush out toxins, heal, create lean muscle bass, and to finally to work optimally on all cylinders.

Together, all of this makes us fearful, unhappy, angry and fatigued individuals. Meanwhile obesity rates are climbing, people are dying and suffering every day from cardiac related illnesses; and then there is diabetes which poses challenges for millions of people. Honestly, maintaining a healthy lifestyle for us is not just about looking good anymore, it's really about surviving.

What's the alternative to making poor health choices? You see it all around you. For many of us, to live into our mid-fifties and not have heart disease, diabetes, or some other health ailment brought on by unhealthy choices, sedentary lifestyle, pollution, stress, and/or poor diet is really a miracle these days.

Today, heart disease and diabetes are America's top two killers. And the crazy thing is - they are both nearly 100% preventable – if not manageable. This is why it is more important than ever to get a hold of your health, but more importantly shift our lifestyles in a new and healthier direction.

Now, many people might assume that they will have to "give up" all of their favorite foods to enjoy their ideal weight and good health. Many diets do that. You have to give up this and that, and never drink this…ah, so many impractical rules! Who can live like that?

Here's the thing, I am not asking you to give up anything! I know what you're thinking: *Huh? **I am not asking you to give up anything.*** Why? *Simply put, this is not a crash diet, it is a lifestyle change.* I am going to ask you to start making better – or different – decisions that you have been to improve your health, lose weight, and feel better.

Okay, to be fair maybe I might be asking you to give up a few things: I am asking you to give up your fatigue, your stress, your poor moods, and feelings of desperation to lose weight. Ultimately, however, the choice is yours. It has always been your choice. Many of us have been fooled into thinking otherwise.

Living the life you want to live may require you to focus more on certain healthy foods over others, but it does not require you to give up every delicious or "sinful" food available. If you think that I have given up some of my favorite foods like ice-cream and the occasional glass of wine, I assure you this is not the case. I still enjoy many of my foods – I just enjoy them in moderation.

The difference now, is that I know where these foods all fit into my meal plan and how I can enjoy them while still maintaining my weight and feeling great. The same goes for you too.

Don't throw in the towel or give up because you think you can't do every single principle, follow every hardcore rule every single day! This is not an all or nothing deal. It is you implementing each principle the best way you can, each and every day - and allowing the changes compound into a sum that is greater than we can imagine.

Are you ready to change your life? I know that I am excited for you and for us to take this journey. Ok, let's get started!

- Taya

Go to
www.totalwellnessbook.com
For FREE tools!

Turn this great book into a wellness support system by downloading templates, documents, recipes and other great tools!

Chapter 1: Goal Setting

Throw everything you have learned about health and fitness out the window. It's time to clear the slate. Clear the deck. Sweep off the floors. Whatever you call it, it's time to start fresh! Chances are you are here because what you have tried in the past just hasn't worked out, right?

That's because many other programs out there simply focus on going to the gym or doing specific exercises or selling you on another lose-weight-fast-scheme. The truth is that looking great and feeling good takes a bit effort, but more importantly it takes consistent effort, which results in a total lifestyle change. Was it always like this? Well, yes and no. Today, we are armed with the more knowledge and scientific evidence, health and fitness education than at any other time in our history. But we are also battling marketing and slick advertising, and chemicals, and hormone-busting preservatives. So, it takes consistent effort to try to see through all the marketing hype and make ourselves better shoppers.

We should never expect to go on a crash diet for three weeks and hope to jump onto a fitness magazine, and afterwards go back to the way we were! It's just not realistic. Being healthy and looking great requires us to change our habits and our routines.

Unfortunately, while many other programs do include the benefits of healthy nutrition, they often don't talk about the real lifestyle choices that are absolutely necessary for us to make in order to achieve the results we want. Perhaps because they don't want to scare people off their new scheme; they don't want to tell people what they really need to hear. So, they provide a bunch of filler with seemingly good sounding advice. But the fact is that it hasn't worked. Diets do not work.

Fitness and nutrition are certainly cornerstones to feeling and looking our very best – and I do spend a lot of time focusing on this throughout my book, but we also require a focus on determining what kind of consumers we are. For example, do we shop in a manner that leads to weight gain? Do we buy healthy foods and healthy products? Could we do better? It's all a learning process, and I hope to help you figure this out.

Let's take me for another example. When I first made the decision to be "totally" healthy, I had to re-evaluate almost everything that I bought at the store from the shampoos and hair conditioners, to make-up products, lotions, and other products that have toxins which we lather, rub, or spray on our bodies. There is no question, that they all have a tremendous impact on our system and health.

This awareness didn't take place overnight. Just like everyone else, I used dozens of harmful products that were sold as "healthy" or as good for me. But as I spent time learning about my health and fitness beyond working out and exercising, I realized that many of us unknowingly make our bodies work harder by the products we buy and by the lifestyle we choose to have.

A Life-Changing Shift is Waiting to Happen

Somewhere deep inside we know that getting into shape and being healthy is good for us. We know that it will help us to feel better, look better, be more productive, and have a better outlook on life. So, why is it such a struggle for so many people?

My years as a personal fitness trainer (and as a student) and time spent with my own personal growth, I struggled with the answer to this question. It is clear that we are often controlled by our habits that we have set in motion many years ago. The way we eat, the way we think about food, and the way we construct our lifestyles all form the basis of which our habits determine the life we have.

Years of indoctrination and years of subtle (and not-so-subtle) marketing by dozens of industries who gain to profit from the rest of us maintaining an un-healthy lifestyle, is hard to overcome on our own. Even our parents and grandparents have been bombarded with advertisements, new products, and fad weight loss diets – all in the name of profit. The downfall was our health, skyrocketing heart disease, diabetes, and other chronic diseases – not to mention cancers of all kinds. Certainly the cause for increasing rates of autism and other conditions in the last twenty years is making us realize that maybe our lifestyle, our choice of foods, and chemicals that we put into our bodies or smear onto our skin, hormones we inject into our foods, unpronounceable food additives, just may have something to these new challenges. The jury may still be out, but I know which direction I am heading in – and it's not your "mainstream" type of thinking.

You see, by being "mainstream" all we get is setting the framework for being fat and struggling with sugar addiction for the rest of our lives. I bet if you are reading this, then you are tired of the "mainstream" way of life and you want to start fresh, new, and feel good again. This requires going against the grain and taking the road less traveled. Let me explain.

Whatever it Takes to Get You Going

Though we sometimes expect a grand parade or something big and uniquely ceremonial about starting a "new healthy life" or making new changes, often times, getting your life and your health on the right track begins with small and *seemingly* insignificant steps, which, taken together, can lead to incredible progress. Sometimes it can be as simple as choosing an apple instead of a candy bar for a snack, taking the stairs, parking further away in the parking lot, walking to the corner store, or simply putting one foot in front of the other and going for a walk. Voila! No grand parade or send off, just the quiet reflection of a decision well-made, followed by another – and another - is sufficient for great change.

In addition, you don't have to wait for arbitrary dates or days to start your new life. You don't have to wait until "after you vacation" or at New Year's Eve. You don't have to wait until Monday or the first of the month. Start today. Start with simple steps.

Often, the gap between intuitively knowing what is good for you and "doing it" is, sometimes feels wider than the Atlantic Ocean. Yet it's great to see just how quickly the gap closes when we take our first step, when we lace our running shoes up, when we close the door behind us as we go out for our evening walk, skip the chip and soda aisle, or when we open the doors and walk into the gym!

Getting serious about our health and fitness can be ultimately transformative in our lives – affecting everything from our moods, health, relationships, to our job performance.

But here's the deal: If you need a ceremony to begin your new life, then do it. If you need to throw out all of your junk food in your pantry in one afternoon, then do it! If you need to buy a new pair of running shoes and workout clothes to get started then do it! If you need to throw out your television set or your comfortable chair that you plop yourself on every time you get home from work to get yourself out and moving, then do it!

Do whatever it takes to get yourself going because once you get going and begin to see the results it's a great feeling and you will want to continue.

Seeing a difference in your life creates a rush that is often hard to replace with anything else! The more you do the better it gets. The body is the only machine that gets better the more you use it. There is nothing quite like seeing improvements in your health and physique when you start off. No doubt, you will be kicking yourself because you wished that you would have started sooner!

We know the following basic equation:

$$\text{Eat healthy} + \text{Exercise More} =$$
$$\text{Equals Better Health.}$$

This book will work with this equation and **then add to it** because we also know that life is much more sophisticated when it comes to our health. Other factors including those influenced by our environment, the products we buy, our stress levels, and our sense of efficacy – that is, our sense of empowerment and our personal fortitude to stay on track through motivation to stay with our goals that we create.

"Eat healthy, exercise more" – we've heard this for a hundred years and yet, the world is getting fatter. We're getting more diseases. We are getting more cancers. We are feeling worse. The slogan sounds great, but it hasn't worked.

Sure, I agree in the number crunching: more calories consumed and the less burned will equal more storage of fat. It's been drilled into us for years. But has it motivated us to move in the direction we want to move in? **The number crunching says no.**

We know that the world is getting fatter. We know that the world is battling chronic diseases like diabetes, obesity, and heart disease. We know that companies are making their chairs bigger for bigger customers and clothes bigger too. We know rates of everything bad – cancer, cholesterol, cortisol, etc. are going up. No, they are skyrocketing.

We know that in a world filled with technology we don't expend a lot of physical energy. Going "with the flow" means ending up overweight and being an excellent candidate to end up with a chronic disease that is largely preventable! We know that going with the grain will end in many of us taking multiple medications, multiple times per day, and feeling worse off for it.

Again, I will say this again: do whatever it is you need to do get yourself going!

Small Steps Make a Huge Difference!

Everything we do has an effect on our health: Getting a small coffee instead of a "Venti" (super-sized) sugar caffeinated drink… an orange, instead of an orange scone or a cup of yogurt instead of sugar-and-preservative rich bowl of ice-cream. All this topped off with a walk after dinner and a plan to do it again – and more – tomorrow is a great start for us. These small changes and decisions make a difference over time and throughout the course of our lives.

How good we are to our bodies in our twenties will affect how we look in our thirties. What we do in our thirties will determine what kind of 40's we will have, and so on. No doubt there are positive long term implications to taking care of ourselves every day.

The good news is that taking care of ourselves today has some pretty good immediate consequences too:

- **We feel better about ourselves**
- **We are able to concentrate better**
- **We sleep better**
- **Our skin and eyes are clearer**
- **We are better able to cope with daily stress**
- **We develop a sense of empowerment**

Really the list can go on and on, but I think you get my point. Making small changes every day leads to radical results in our health and fitness overtime.

We have to be aware that we are constantly battling "instant gratification" syndrome that we have grown accustomed to. We are a culture that wants things right now – we want instant results, we want instant satisfaction. Small and effective decisions will not make you drop 20 pounds by tomorrow morning. We need to keep things into perspective and stay focused – our attitude will help with that.

We all know that smoking cigarettes is bad for us, but did you know that there is some emerging research that now argues that having a sedentary lifestyle can be much worse than actually smoking cigarettes? It's true. What we do every single day matters! Taking small steps every day, several times a day, all adds up!

Whenever you are feeling discouraged, whenever you are feeling down about where you are at, consider the healthy choices you can make right then to change your mood. Can you take a walk? Can you go for a bike ride? Can you make a healthy meal? Can you spend time in meditation? Do you see how every small thing is a part can add up to sum much bigger than you can imagine. Taking several small steps today can put the brakes on the direction you are heading towards.

Deciding to move forward right then with a small and *seemingly insignificant choice* is powerful! The truth is that every choice we make towards a healthy life is significant.

Nobody Likes To Do Chores

As I will discuss further in this book, our mental focus and attitude also matters significantly with regards to our progress over time. It's the "over time" that usually stumps people. It's the "over time" that usually separates those who will see results and those who will end up back on their sofas or love seats that they should have thrown out.

If you want to see change in your life, you will have to make small, but tough decisions – every day. To sustain ourselves "over time" we have to make our exercise regimen and our "eating" habits, anything but routine. We have to destroy the concept of exercise or healthy cooking as a "chore." When we pigeon hole our exercise or food preparation into a chore it immediately triggers negative connotations in our mind. We tend to lose focus, interest, and ultimately handle it differently.

Remove from your mind frame that the exercises you do are part of your daily "chores." Remove from your mental landscape that "cooking healthy" is boring or hard. Your new lifestyle is anything but a chore, but **rather a choice** that you are happy to make.

A chore is something that you have to do, often because you are forced to do so. A choice – even difficult choices – honor a sense of ownership to the direction you are taking. Make your healthy life a lifestyle choice and not a chore!

To make your fitness and healthy eating habits anything but a chore, add diversity, color, and purpose into every exercise and every meal. The minute you feel like you are "falling" into a routine, jolt things a bit. Try some new exercise, walk a different way back home, search for a few new recipes, shop at a different health food store, join a new club, or reach out and make new and positive friends. Do whatever you have to do to maintain your priorities and focus. I enjoy training with several close friends, but I also like to take on new clients and train with other experts in my field. Doing so adds a little fresh blood in the mix and keeps me motivated and sharp. Consider adding a new work out buddy, a new walking partner, or someone you can be active with.

Making Tough Choices

Chances are we all probably have a favorite TV show and while we may take some time to watch it, what do we do after? We probably keep the television on to watch something else that we don't like or sort of like. Soon, two or three hours have passed and probably a countless amount of calories and sugar consumed by snacking – because many of us like to snack when we watch TV.

Many of our "empty" calories that we take in are consumed on autopilot. We finished off that bowl of chips because it was in front of us. You ate the rest of the desert because you got really into the movie and wanted to "munch" on something. You ordered the whopping plate of fried onion rings, fries, and dip because you wanted to stay for another round of beer... the list is endless.

But what if knew this weakness and turned it around? What if we made simple choices that prevented us from going down that unhealthy road? And, what if we did this every day – or even weekly? What if we had a taken 30 minutes to stretch, go for a walk, and plan out our meals for the week while we were watching our television show? Or better yet what if we left to television off turned off and exercised or spent quality time with our family at the park?

To be sure we need to make tough choices. But the more tough choices we make the more progress we will generate! In a little bit, I will be discussing shopping – how we shop for food and products also impacts our total weight, fitness, and overall health. We can't deny this big white elephant in the room: how we shop affects our health.

If you show me someone's fridge and pantry, ninety-nine times out of a hundred, I will tell you if you he or she is fat or not.

Looking Beyond the "Fat" Problem

We get up in the morning walk past our mirror and focus on our problem area. We pinch our fat and we turn half way around focus on the spot that we want to get rid of. You've done this. We have ALL done this. We sigh and try to figure out a way to address it by maybe getting a diet soda for lunch and then we're right back where we started the next morning in front of the mirror!

But what if we try something different? What if we focused on our body in a different manner? What if we looked beyond the fat? What if instead of focusing on the problem we focus a little more on the solution?

What we have been doing all along just isn't working. We have to look beyond the fat. The answer to our problem lies beyond where we have been scammed into to reaching.

In his NY Times best-selling book, *Does This Clutter Make My Butt Look Fat?,* author Peter Walsh believes that our fat problem and weight issues as a culture, is a mere symptom of something larger. The North American culture of consumption, over-eating, and "can't get enough of anything" attitude, which holds dear to the notion that "more is better" and bigger is better, all fuels our consumption for bigger homes, bigger cars, the need for bigger storage lockers, and the need of having bigger chairs, so that our bigger butts can be more comfortable! (3)

Ironically, we know this. We understand this. But we go along with the crowd anyway. Why? A majority of us simply can't stop ourselves. We need bigger chairs, bigger plates, bigger drinks, bigger portions, bigger garages, bigger cars, and bigger stomachs because we just can't get enough. We can't consume fast enough. We are constantly overwhelmed by the bigger lives we create for ourselves. We are drowning in big!

But we know this deep down in our minds and hearts. We see ourselves getting fatter. And it wreaks havoc on our emotions and our sense of empowerment.

So our response? To buy more and eat more! Yikes! Now it becomes a never ending cycle of poor choices that results in getting us (that is me and you) fatter, less healthy, and unable to achieve what we really want to achieve in life. At the end of the day we don't feel better about ourselves. We know that this is unsustainable, but we don't know how to stop. Humans often gravitate towards the path of least resistance. We're wired to avoid pain. Our brains are wired to seek out calorie-rich and fatty foods because long ago, food was often scarce. That reality is long gone.

It's More Expensive to Be Overweight

There is no question that being overweight and unhealthy is expensive and hard on our budgets. Take for account our lost days of work and productivity because of being sick, doctor office visits, more blood work, daily medications prescribed, and the cost of more unhealthy junk food and beverages.

In his book, *Does This Clutter Make My Butt Look Fat,* Peter Walsh argues that clutter doesn't give us enough room to breathe and to deal with the priorities we need to deal with to get healthy. He argues that the first steps to effective weight loss entail "decluttering" our mind and our homes – and our lifestyles. Clutter like fat are often synonymous with each other. "The clutter didn't appear overnight and won't disappear overnight," he writes.

Walsh, a professional "declutterer" writes that when he first works with people in their homes, he doesn't focus on what people should throw away or recycle. He first focuses on what matters. I like that idea. It coincides with how I feel about health and fitness. For us to have the health and body we want, we too, need to look beyond our fat and our problem areas, and actually focus on what we really want. We need to focus on what matters. (4)

Consider what Walsh writes: "Your food. Your career. Your relationships. Your schedule. Your buying habits. Your diet. Consider for a moment that where you live, what you own, how you interact with others, what you eat, and how you spend your time. These are all intimately linked. You can't change one piece without affecting all the others. Declutter your mind, declutter your home, declutter your relationship to food. Then watch the ripple effect this has on every aspect of your life," writes Walsh. (5)

From my personal and professional experience, I can certainly agree with him. Our ability to be successful in our goals is founded on our ability to focus on the real goal, and not the problem. It makes sense, so why are we focused on the problem? Because it's an easier distraction and easier to visualize – it's already in front of us. We see it. We feel it. We think about it every day.

As modern-day humans, we often focus on the negatives. Did you know that if you received ninety-nine (that's 99) wonderful complements and receive only one (1) negative comment today, I want you to guess which comment that you will focus on when you go to bed tonight? 99% of the time, we will focus on that one single negative comment.

Walsh is right, we need to declutter our minds, our lives, and make the necessary room for change. If you want change, you better be ready to let go of some essential unhealthy habits you have been living with.

Thinking Beyond the Weight Loss

Sometimes our health issues lie beyond "weight loss." In order for us to be successful at achieving the kind of fitness goals we want, we shouldn't focus on the "fat" or the "the problem" but our goal – our vision.

Most certainly, the ability to address our weight loss and fitness goals in our lives relies on our ability to be honest with ourselves. And the chances are that if you picked up this book, you are ready to move forward. Most of the diets and fitness books out there focus on not what we want, but what we don't want – belly fat, love handles, and fatigue, etc.

In his book, Walsh also discusses some important points as to why we often fail and that I would like to share, namely, we have become a culture of excuse-making people. I know that this might be difficult at first to hear. But when we stop to examine that correct observation and let it sink in – we realize that he is right. As a culture, we are absolutely wonderful at making up excuses.

Let's delve into his thinking a bit further when it comes to his argument: The first excuse, which I have personally used before, is: "I simply don't have the time to do what it takes to get to my goal."

"I don't have the time..." I know that our lives can be busy. We all have to learn to balance what we want with what's important – bills, job, parental responsibilities, fun, time with family, and exercise – etc. It is easy to tell ourselves that we simply don't have the time. In fact, who can argue with that, right? Nearly everyone is leading chaotic, cluttered, and unhealthy lives.

We often place exercise and our healthy as the last thing we do – if we have time. If I had more time, I would eat better. If I had more time, I would learn about ingredients more. If I had more time, I would prepare and cook my meals healthier. If had more time, I would walk – instead of drive - to the corner store. If I had more time, I would write down what I've eaten during the day. **"If I only had more time!" We say that so many times, that in turn, it becomes the dialogue of our life's story.**

All these decisions impact our health, in one way or another. They are all small but important decisions that affect our personal culture, our habits, and our feelings about who we are. We simply need to make more time. What we need however, is to create more time by getting rid of a lot of clutter in our lives.

The unfortunate thing is we spend so much time thinking about our fat, our problem spots, and our state of health that we don't even recognize it. Then, we turn around and give ourselves the ultimate excuse no one can argue with: we just don't have the time.

In reality we do have the time. We spend so much time dieting, looking at ourselves in the mirror, slouched on the couch, or feeling sorry for ourselves, which all takes up our time too!

Another Big Fat Excuse We Tell Ourselves:

Nothing will work for me; I'm a lost cause... Oh boy, this argument suggests that change really needs to happen way down with our sense of empowerment before we can move forward. Sometimes, people give up long before they try because of their defeated attitude.

Have you ever told yourself this: "I have tried to be healthy, and it simply doesn't work, so why bother?" If you are like most people, at some point, you probably have had this internal conversation and so, you give up long before you get started. But there is a morsel of truth in there!

Dieting for the "short term" doesn't work. The fact is that you have tried (many times) and of course these diets – every last one of them – have failed you. I like the way Walsh describes it: "Dieting doesn't work. Have you ever met someone who used to be fat but conquered the problem long ago? That person probably doesn't say, 'I've been on a diet for ten years.' She says, 'I learned how to eat.' Think of it this way: If you your new eating plan succeeds, it's a change in your life. If it fails, it's a diet." (6)

In my years of experience as a personal trainer, I have seen dozens, if not hundreds, of popular diets come and go. I never liked the idea of a "diet" because they are often fleeting, they are temporary, and they are certainly not the long term answer for you or me.

In my opinion however, they fill an important void that is generated by a culture who wants instant gratification, instant results, and easy weight loss at the drop of the hat without much effort. We can't seriously expect to go on some type of "lemon and honey diet" (or whichever is the diet craze today) and expect to wake up tomorrow looking a like a fitness model! Our bodies don't work that way. Life doesn't work that way. Yet, time and time again we have expected it to.

Trainers and doctors are often in a similar situation with this regard: It's not uncommon for people eat hamburgers, fries, and drink beers and smoke cigars every week for forty years and then expect to be fit after one doctor's visit! In this marketing-dominated culture we have been sold that we can have everything we want – including perfect health and fitness – fast and easy – despite our unhealthy way of life.

The truth is that diets will not get you where you want to go for two reasons: they are temporary and they don't focus on what you want, but instead they focus on what you don't want.

Let me explain this a bit further:

Diets are temporary: Most diets, even some diets that I find appealing for a variety of reasons are too restrictive to be a "life-long" way of eating. I don't think that while exercising and planning your meals, you should be juicing for three weeks, going on a watermelon diet for seven days, or going without the right kind of carbohydrates for the rest of your life.

Demonizing whole swaths of food categories just doesn't make sense. Diets are always circling around the latest trends, the latest fruit craze, or the latest supplement discovery, in hopes to show off the "next big thing," and to use lingo that we are comfortable with: No carbs, No Fats, No This, No That. These are diets never really meant to succeed in the long-term.

Heavily restricting your diet is not only bad for your health, increases weight gain in the long run, leaves you feeling depressed and fatigued, but often times it tears into your muscles, which is what we don't want. In fact, thank Goodness diets are temporary!

Focusing on the wrong thing: Diets are particularly good at telling you all the things you can't eat: Don't eat this, don't eat that. In fact, I think there are a few books and magazines that are very popular with a similar title. Diets focus on temporary "weight loss" schemes developed more by marketers than fitness experts – when we really should be focusing on total health – our stress levels, our lifestyle, the products we buy, etc.

Fat and unhealthy is the easiest thing to be in North America.

Becoming fat is the easiest thing you can do in today's culture, according to Walsh. And I agree. In fact, you don't have to even try. You can eat till your heart explodes, watch TV until your butt gets bigger, and take a pill when it gets too much to get out of your chair. "Going with the flow" is what Walsh calls it in his book. If you want to be fit, if you want to be healthy, if you want to look and feel great, then you will have to go against the current. And I'm in total agreement.

Most of us do simply go with flow. I say "most" of us, because a majority of us have a problem with our weight. We say, "Yes" to pretty much anything that will make our lives easier and satisfy us immediately: Supersize your breakfast, lunch, or dinner? Yes! Another round of beers? Yes! Do you want a party-size bag of potato chips? Should we drive to visit friends down the block? Yes! You get my drift here, right? Yes!

We live in a culture that says "yes" to nearly everything, except our fitness and long term health goals. We say yes to more consumption, more fat, and more feelings of regret and despair when we receive the bill that comes at the end of the party. But what if we said "No" every once in a while? Or what if we said "No" just 70% of the time? Would we save a few calories? Would we save a few dollars?

The chances are that if we thought about our consumption we would save quite a bit over the course of a week, a month, a year, and a lifetime!

Our Relationship With Food Matters

Sometimes we eat and we just don't know why. Sometimes we'll put on a movie and not realize that we just finished a whole bag of sodium. We've all been there. We might not have even liked what we've been eating!

We simply eat, just to eat! Sometimes we eat because we are sad, upset, angry, lonely, bored, or fearful. We often have seemingly "natural" tendency to do so because we've a good portion of us have been conditioned to except food as a reward or prize for being good.

Something in our brains and in our vision for how we want to live has to overcome this urge to eat "just to eat." Deep down, we know this. We know that we probably should not eat that entire tub of ice-cream because we are sad, or had a bad day at work. This small "failure" rolls downhill like an avalanche. We give up on our budding healthy habits and skid out control back towards our old way of life of being unfit and unhealthy.

It's hard for many of us to escape this simple truth: we have an emotional connection with food. It is there for us every day. It is not only essential for life, but it becomes essential for our moods. How many of us have eaten food, because we were bored? How many of us ate food just because it was just there? Or how many of us eat popcorn, candy, and drink soda at the movies, because well, that is what we do at the movies? This leads me to my next important point to consider: triggers.

Triggers for Food

We all have triggers that spark particular behaviors. You pull out a cigarette when you start drinking with buddies. You have a cookie every time you get a mocha or soy latte. You grab your favorite ice cream when you watch your favorite television shows for three hours a night. These are all triggers. Many times we do this unconsciously. Our triggers become our habits. Our habits become the building blocks of our lifestyle.

To eliminate the things that widen the gap between our goal and where we are today, we need to focus on our "triggers." Pay attention to them. This simple act of acknowledging the triggers that result in certain behavior is powerful. In fact, it brings the triggering act from the "subconscious" level to the "conscious" level.

Once we recognize what we are going, and why we are doing it, we are often in a better situation to ignore it or replace it with something healthier. We need to stop pulling these triggers! There are some triggers that we can replace rather easily after we figure them out.

For example, if you only smoke cigarettes when you drink beers with your buddies, what would you do it you stopped drinking beers? Or what if you substitute drinking beers with another non-alcoholic beverage?

You could be eliminating two birds with one stone – or two potentially triggering mechanism with one healthy, consistent choice.

By identifying and confronting our triggers, we are able to effectively build new healthier habits. Over time, these healthier habits translate to healthier bodies, real weight loss, and feelings of empowerment.

Remember, if we want to see real changes, then we are going to have to bite the bullet and make some real changes in our lives! Making these changes isn't always easy. If they were, then there would be hard bodies walking up and down the street.

There is certainly a silver lining here. We can also use these mechanisms for positive triggers as well. For example, we can create a trigger that every time we have dinner, we go for a short walk afterwards. Every meal triggers a healthy walk, instead of a cigarette. Even during our lunch break at work we can take time to eat healthy meal and take a short walk. We can create dozens of healthy triggers to replace the negative ones!

A Complete Holistic Path of Health & Fitness

A total fitness book wouldn't do anyone justice if we focused solely on fitness and nutrition without talking about the chemical and hormonal effects that are caused by the items and products we purchase at the grocery store. It would be like the old saying: taking one step forward and two steps back! The chemicals that we expose ourselves to every day (sunscreen, lotions, cosmetics, etc.) actually work against us in our effort for optimal health.

No doubt, we need to think about not just eating lean protein, organic fruits and vegetables but we also need to focus on our general lifestyle choices, purchasing decisions, and stress levels, in order to maintain and sustain excellent health.

But how do we get there? After all, we all want to look and feel great, right? We all have a desire to look and feel our best, but why do so many of us fail to reach even a fraction of our potential? Usually, it is because we forget to establish clear and reachable goals for ourselves.

The idea of setting goals is something we're all familiar with. Whether are goal is to finish college, buy a home, or learn how to play the piano, our goals play an important role in our lives and the success we experience.

Goals Often Arise from Deep within Us

The ability to see our goals manifest is often a personal and worthy venture which offers us the ability to feel fulfilled and content with our lives. Other times, our goals are simply passing thoughts or desires that eventually turn into something real, tangible, and visual. When we set goals for improving our health and fitness, we are able to take real and consistent steps to reach those goals. Unfortunately, sometimes our fitness and health goals lead to failure. However, our efforts don't have to end in failure.

What I have found is that the first step to successfully achieving our goals is to determine the question of "Why?" For example, why do you want to get into better shape? Do you have an event or occasion that you want to look your best at? Do you want to combat stress, sleep, and feel better? Maybe you want to create fresh and healthier outlook and body image?

Knowing what the reason is that you have set this goal in the first place will help you to stay on track. The goals we create often arise deep within us. They tug at our hearts. We speak softly to us when we take time to listen. If we grab on to those goals and do our best to make sure they manifest, the success is often much closer than we realize.

The Secret Why Most Diets Don't Work

Do you know why don't most diets work? Let's cut right to the chase. The reason is simple. Most diets trigger what's called a "famine response" that get people in trouble for many years after they make a decision to lose weight by severely restricting their calorie intake with any particular diet.

Never heard of the "famine response"? Let me illustrate the point further. When we catch a cold or pick up a virus, our bodies naturally create antibodies. For our bodies, this is a natural response to fight off any future attack. Similarly, our bodies have a natural response to periods of famine.

So what is a "famine response" and how does it happen?

Most diets call for a severe restriction in calories, which is normal for dieting. But since consumers demand quick action, diets usually begin to restrict their calories right away. After a couple of weeks of severe calorie restriction the body sheds weight pretty fast. The people dieting think this is great and so do the diet producers – who can then claim that their diets work. But what happens after several months? While all these changes are taking place outside out bodies, just below the surface, your brain and your body is beginning to react to that severe restriction of calories, and it does so by triggering a "famine response." When your body begins to think that there is a famine – or a lack of food – it does a couple of things – it slows down your metabolism and it makes it more difficult for you to lose weight.

After you get back on a "normal" diet, your body gains that weight back very quickly. What's worse is that it becomes harder and harder to lose that weight again with the same routine or calorie restriction because our body makes it more difficult to unlock those precious storage reserves we call fat.

So, what do we usually do to get results? We elect to go on an even stricter diet and again shock our system into another famine response. But shortly after that, you gain the weight back! The cycle continues. There are many names for this, but this "Yo-Yo" dieting happens to many, many people on many popular weight loss diets and in the end does not help our fitness and health goals at all. **My question is:** Aren't you ready to leave behind the "Yo-Yo" diets behind?

When you are participating on the latest "fad diet," your body is thinking, "Hey, there is no more food out there, so anything I get a hold of I will then store away (into fat), and throw away the key. Nope, I will not let this fat go - never!" If I wanted to lose weight, why would I cause my body to react like this? Sadly, millions create this same response in their own body every single day.

Diets Create an Even Larger Problem Later

In effect, many diets, in the long run, make it easier for you to gain weight and harder for you to lose the fat! So, the cycle begins again. In order to lose more weight, we do even crazier things submit to even ridiculous levels of dieting, to lose a pound. But like a springboard, soon after it brings us deeper into despair, more weight gain, and even health problems. This exactly what you do not want to happen! Your body remembers every calorie restriction period, known as the "famine" period. This will forever make it more difficult for you to lose weight.

This is fairly common knowledge. But take on and entertain these fad diets anyway. We focus explicitly on the "numbers" and forget about the rational way to lead a healthy life. To be sure, if you are a professional body builder, athlete, or trainer, you will focus and complete and total health and wellness as a part of your training. Everything you do – from your eating habits, sleep hygiene, training, and your lifestyle affects your performance.

Why People Fail at Real Weight Loss

If you are watching a professional skier, basketball player, or ballet dancer, you are watching someone who put in thousands upon thousands of hours of work to make what they do look easy and effortless.

Dedication, sacrifice, and determination create big enough barriers for even the most well intended people. The gap between good intentions (i.e. New Years' Resolutions and starting a new diet) and lofty goals of weight loss and looking great, is often unmatched by the amount of investment that is needed to reach those goals. So, while we might want to "lose" weight and fit into our college jeans, which is often possible, we fail because we don't put in the work that is required to achieve that.

But why is that? After all, it's not that we don't try to get in shape. Sometimes we set ourselves for failure right of the starting gate! We simply don't examine where we are presently, so we actually don't know where to even begin!

Have you ever visited an amusement park and looked a directory map they have posted up to find your way around? If you were trying to find a restroom, a particular ride, or even the exit, the first thing we need to determine is where we are, right?

It sounds a bit obvious, but when it comes to our fitness, many people simply fail because they wander around without a plan, without a goal, and without any real strategy – and without knowing where they are! Soon, they find themselves giving up. The lesson here: To get to where we're going, we need to first find out where we are! This also holds true when we first figure out our path to total wellness.

Why People Succeed with Their Health Goals

People often succeed when they determine where they want to be. But the process also is determined by figuring out exactly where they are, what their vision is, and the realistic bite-size steps to get there. Being aware of our weaknesses is also essential and just as part of the mix as any other element to success.

For example, a championship team may not have the best offense (their scoring capabilities might be a weaknesses) so by employing methods to "shore up" and strengthen their weakness and even utilizing their strength of playing excellent defense they still can compete and win.

People succeed because they have made a choice to first determine where they are – what are their positives and their weaknesses lie and then move towards their goals with a better of understanding of their capabilities.

As we move forward in this book, we will continuously touch on the topic of success in our daily lives and in achieving the health and fitness we want.

Assessing Where You Are Now

In every aspect of our lives, we all have to start somewhere. Whether we want to climb out of financial debt or if we want to get in better shape, we need to first determine where we are and find the best path to getting where we want to go. There is no one single right pathway to getting where we want to go. In addition, there is no exact finish line to be crossed. We are striving instead to reach a healthy place where a healthy lifestyle exists.

For starters, I always recommend always visiting your doctor and getting a physical medical examination, your routine blood work, and then getting your doctor's approval for you to start your program.

While we often focus our assessment on the pounds we shed or the inches off the waist that we lose - or even how much weight we can bench press. We also need to consider a more holistic view of our health.

That while we may lose weight and inches, and also gain strength and endurance, we need to consider other important health factors. Some of these essential medical factors your doctor can help you with, such as your level of cholesterol, blood pressure, etc.

In addition, other health factors such as smoking, excessive consumption of alcohol, or getting enough sleep are all important to address in our lives. By reducing the use of cigarettes, alcohol, and getting restful sleep alone, we will see a positive and dramatic impact on our motivational levels, our moods, and our achievements.

So, while you might also want to fit back into your jeans you wore back in college, another very worthy and significant goal would also mean our ability to be "healthy" in general; in addition to such goals as reducing our body fat percentage and increasing our level of endurance, strength, and energy to go along with it. Once we have taken the time to assess our situation, we need to create our own personal vision, which will guide us through our journey to better health.

I want to emphasize "personal" vision. Since we can't simply adopt someone else's vision. There is no one size fits all. Your vision is closely tied to your spiritual and emotional place in the world. It is through your vision, your personal vision, where you will generation your inner strength.

My Initial Assessment of Those I Train & Work With

There are a series of questions I ask all of my clients during our initial assessment. For example, I would start by asking them what their ultimate goal is and how committed they are to it. In addition, before we begin, I ask them what they currently do or have done in the past for exercise. I also ask them what their lifestyle is like. Are they generally active? What is their schedule like? Have they been ill recently? What is the general state of their health? Are there any past, recent, and potentially problematic health factors, such as injuries?

Before our first session, I also ask them to bring a food journal which consists of three days of everything they have eaten, which would include how much water they drink, coffee, alcohol, etc. It is also important for me to know if they have any injuries or limitations. Also, it's very important that I know what medications they are taking (if any) and whether they have any medical problems.

You really need to know what you are starting with to devise an appropriate plan. Certainly, when I start training with someone, the person's current health, commitment level, and how they currently feel about their body image is very important.

I have had some pretty stubborn clients who automatically want to cut calories when losing weight for summer or events that they have limited time to get ready for. I get tons of people coming to me asking how they can lose weight fast! Unfortunately, I am the one who usually has to provide a reality check for some of my clients. Often, they look at me surprised at my words. But how could we be surprised? After all, we are inundated by marketing that hides the truth: Losing weight and looking great requires a commitment that we don't expect.

Realistically with proper diet and exercise you can lose 4 - 8 lbs. of fat per month. For a beginner, you can gain about 3 lbs. of muscle per month but tapers off after a few months. You want to make sure your goals are S.M.A.R.T which stands for Specific, measurable, Attainable, Realistic, Timely. Avoid setting yourself up for failure! The first time I meet with a client after getting to know them we start with setting realistic goals and coming up with a plan of action.

Once we understand the initial assessment, we begin to create our vision and find our focus point. Having a vision is essential to our success. Not only does it help us stay focused but it helps to sustain ourselves when we are in the "valleys" and feel like giving up.

I also ask them to detail for me what their goals are. Many people tell me, "Well, I just want to get in shape!" or "I want to lose a few pounds." What I try to do is get them to break things down into specific goals: such as I want to lose 20 pounds within 4 months, etc. Being specific about our goals allows us to better focus our attention on what it's going to take to get there. Much of that starts out with our ability to determine what our vision is.

Creating Your Vision

Having a vision is so important to our success in anything we do, including increasing our fitness and carving out a healthier lifestyle. Our vision is a mental and emotional reflection of what the future that we believe could exist. Our vision will lead to creating manageable goals and our ultimate success.

But how do we create our vision?

There is no right or wrong way in creating a person vision. Each of us has different mental and emotional backgrounds by which to create our own effective and purposeful vision. With that said, there are a few things you should consider:

Vision is future oriented. Vision incorporates all of our beliefs, hopes, and dreams together. So when we create our vision we need think big – very big. Our vision is where we stretch our faith in whatever direction we choose to go. When it comes to our vision, we are the sole limiting factor. Perhaps it's a good idea to take of the leash and let your vision run wild for a bit, see where it takes you.

To create our vision, we need to ask ourselves what kind of future we want. The process will help to facilitate goal setting and planning. It helps you stay focused. In addition, your vision will help to unleash a powerful desire to move forward.

Like a fingerprint, a vision is always unique and always personal. It entails the essence of the future. So my vision for my life is always going to be different for your life. Respecting each other's vision is paramount and is very important to distinguish in our lives. For me, vision is an intimate concept and requires us to be genuine for us to realize that vision we placed in front of us.

Instituting The Law of Attraction with Weight Loss

I am a true believer in the "Law of Attraction." This simple but powerful law states that we attract that which we are attracted to. In other words *we attract into our lives* whatever we focus our attention on. It can be an extremely useful tool in our daily lives in getting what we want. The beginning starts with having a clear vision for ourselves. (7)

At its essence, the *Law of Attraction* depends much on our vision, our attitude, and our internal conversation that we have about our lives, our goals, our health, and our careers – as you can imagine, the list goes on. Whatever dominates our thinking, dominates our vision, and dominates that which we put our faith into, will often manifest itself into our reality.

We need to take another step of faith once we've reached this conclusion – we need to create goals – reachable goals to get there. Once we open ourselves up to this level of awareness and consciousness, we begin to see things we often have missed before. We become more focuses, observant, and move forward in life with a grander, more fulfilling sense of purpose.

More Brainstorming & The Law of Attraction

Brainstorming is a part of the whole process of being healthy, looking, and feeling good. Empowering ourselves with the **Law of Attraction** requires us to have a vision – something to focus our energy on.

People brainstorm in a variety of ways. The essential result of brainstorming is to extract all the potential ideas out of your inside, whether they are from your heart or your mind. Getting down on paper (or your computer) is helpful, because you can save it. This is the basic difference between brainstorm and daydreaming.

A Vision Board Exercise:

Take a walk by yourself and allow yourself to daydream about being healthy, being in better shape, of feeling better. Think about what you want to see realized in say, a year or five years. Is it losing 10 or

30 pounds? Is it getting off your high-blood pressure medication? Is it being able to do a particular activity?

Visualize yourself doing this. Allow yourself to dream and think and focus on the minute details of your dreams. When your brain gets going, you will find competing thoughts kicking around. That's okay. Allow yourself the time to continue focusing on your vision until becomes clearer.

When you are finished with your walk, either sit down in front of your computer or simply get a notebook out and start writing down the thoughts that have managed to stay at the forefront of your mind. When you are done, take a minute to look and think about what you had written down. Keep track of your progress.

Next we are going to create a vision board. This is simply a board that has photos and other visuals of your dreams and your vision. Print out or cut out what you have written down and consider attaching a few pictures it. (You might consider doing an internet search on vision boards to help you!)

Do you want to wear the same clothes or be as fit as you were in high school or college? Place these pictures or others on your vision board. Attach headlines that break down your ultimate vision and place them on your board. If you don't find any headlines that fit, simply create your own.

Your vision is a fluid set of ideas, thoughts that you are never fully "done" with. So, in essence, your vision board is also always evolving. Nevertheless, once you are satisfied with it place up in your office, kitchen, or someplace that you are sure to see it every morning.

Coming up with a Realistic plan for YOU

We are only here because of you. It's you that we need to pay attention to right now. Coming up with a plan that works for you is essential to your success. Now that our vision is more clearly defined, now that you have brainstormed, and created your vision board, it's time to create a realistic plan. I will offer some realistic examples by which you can measure and track your progress. In addition, coming up with measurable goals and real "benchmarks" to establish a method of tracking your progress can help.

Essentially, a realistic plan entails something that you can manage. If you can't measure it, then you can't manage it. So, consider the following:

Tracking Your Progress

Tracking my progress really helps me to stay motivated. You don't need to track your progress to get results but I find the more I see the progress on paper the more excited I am to keep going. Also with any goal whether fitness or something else, the better able you are to look at your progression over time.

The bigger the goal the more important it is to set mini-goals and milestones and reach a satisfying place to "check off" the specific benchmarks as you accomplish them. Consider setting up some goals and also instituting a reward system when you reach each one!

The more organized you are the better your plan will follow course. You will also be able to tell if something is working for you or if you need to make changes. I am a big fan of the Charles Poliquin "Bio Signature Test," because it will tell you what your body fat percentage is, which is what I find the most accurate way to track your progress.

Interestingly, there is a trainer named Ryan Herszkowicz who works in downtown Toronto who first introduced me to it. After being impressed with my own experience with it, I now request all my clients to get tested with him initially and then every 4 weeks following. The results have been pretty amazing.

Tracking your results can be extremely motivating and keep you focused!

Let's say that among other changes in your life, you are going to not worry about the weight you are going to lose, but rather use something a bit more concrete in terms of tracking your progress. Your "weight" can actually fluctuate throughout the day and throughout the week, so consider your weekly average as a way to consistently weight yourself over time.

So, let's say that you want to track your progress using other variables. You decide that you are going to use time (days) against which you will measure your progress. So, every four weeks you will track your progress to make sure you are not hitting a plateau.

We consistently write down the amount of time we are spending doing a particular exercise – it can be walking, cycling, jogging, or doing crunches. You want to make note of the time and the distance traveled.

Why does this matter? These numbers don't mean anything to anyone except you. These are your personal best times. So, consider that by tracking progress comparing one day to the next, we will be able to find an average for a particular week. Track your daily and weekly averages. Are you improving your time? Is it taking you a shorter amount of time to walk three miles or cycle ten miles? If you want to get a bit more into specifics for your goals, consider tackling a 30 day, 60 day, or even a 90 day goal. Let's examine this further now.

Use the following to fill in your numbers:

My current weight/measurements: _____

- **30 day goal: _____**
- **60 day goal: _____**
- **90 day goal: _____**

Are these realistic goals? How do you know if you are underestimating or over estimating yourself? Often, we won't know until we try, right? Like I said, there is no right or wrong way here. Whatever it takes? Do you need to alter your goal slightly after several attempts? That's fine. Just make sure that the goal is challenging enough for you to ensure your progress.

Holding yourself Accountable (Creating Measurable Benchmarks)

Like anything else, you need to be able to write out your goals and check your progress. Simply, "tracking it in your head" will not do! We all know that life can get overwhelming and thoughts can crowd out our focus. Holding yourself accountable entails physically tracking your progress in some way – either by using a notebook, computer software program, or smart phone application. Consider also getting a "workout" buddy that will be able to check on you and your progress.

Do you remember when I stated before, that you need to do "whatever it takes?" Well that includes now. You need to do whatever it takes for you get this done. Tracking your progress is critical for you to maintain your path and your movement forward.

Writing things down where you see them every day, increases your sense of ownership and obligation. It helps us prioritize. Life has a way of pushing things aside, especially if they are inconvenient. What if we flipped the equation around? What if we made everything else less convenient and our work out priority? How more successful would we be at reaching our goals?

Helpful Recommendations

There is no right way or wrong way to keep yourself motivated. However, there are a few things that work. You can consider, putting photo's up of people with fit bodies (including yourself at a younger age); write down your progress in a journal, take before and after photos. And of course, creating, developing, and adding to your vision board. If you have experience success and achievement in the face of adversity, you know that the battle is always won and lost in our mind. Doing whatever it takes to keep your mind focused on your goals is well worth your time and effort.

- **Put up photos of yourself**
- **Use a vision board**
- **Use a workout journal consistently**
- **Keep yourself accountable to a friend**

Creating a Sustainable Mindset for the Long Haul

For some people exercise and proper nutrition can be a huge life style change and it can be quite overwhelming. Getting into shape requires your efforts to be consistent. Start by setting aside days/times for your workouts and commit to them, no excuses!

Start by building your workouts into your daily schedule and weekly calendar. We all have to make time to eat, sleep, shower, right? Embedding your consistent exercise routine within your schedule promotes consistency.

When we build our exercise and health routine in to our schedule, instead of making it an "extra" we take ourselves to a higher level of achievement. Our exercise and health routine doesn't just become an occasional "event" but rather a habit that we cannot do without.

Consider Five Easy Things You Can Do Today to Support Natural Weight Loss

While many of us struggle with weight loss, we often gravitate towards "fast weight loss" diets and solutions. While we can drop several pounds pretty quickly with some of these fad diets, we know that most of that weight is the result of a loss of water.

Real and natural weight loss takes a little longer, but it is sustainable and longer lasting. The problem is that many of us don't have the patience to follow through with some simple changes. The fact is that even the simplest, not intrusive lifestyle changes can have positive net results in our lives.

Consider the next five principles for simple things we can to every day to help us lose weight. Some of them sound simple, however many people don't do them. And yet, it's not so much the action itself but the mental mind-frame and perspective that really matter.

In no particular order, they are:

Principle One

When eating, do nothing else. We have a horrible relationship with food in North America. We tend to eat without thinking about what we put in our mouths. Our forks and spoons act like small shovels as we quickly consume our fatty and sugary diets – often without tasting or even chewing it! It's not sustainable, it's not healthy, and it triggers our body to eat more and be satiated less.

The act of eating and actually tasting our foods are one of the best pleasures in our life. Why would we want to hurry through it like a chore? Food is meant to be enjoyed, savored and appreciated. When eating, do nothing else except think about the food you are enjoying. Don't watch television. Don't do homework. Don't eat and drive. Don't eat standing up. Don't eat and check your email or the news of the day on your favorite website. Enjoy your food without doing anything else.

Allow yourself to enjoy your meal, slowly. Too often we spend our time treating our food and our "eating" time like it is something that we just need to get done. When we zip through our food, we take the thought out of it, we lessen our attention, we cheat ourselves out of a healthy relationship with food.

Principle Two
Before Taking Another Bite...Swallow. Before

eating or taking another bite, make sure that the first bite you take is completely done and swallowed. This is a very simple concept that allows you to make sure that you chew your food properly for better digestion. Also this helps you enjoy your food much more effectively. Some people suggest taking a bit and putting your fork or spoon down on the table. This will help you ensure that you are pausing long enough to really chew your food. Sounds strange, right? We're not used to eating this way. However, when you enjoy your food – everyone wins!

Sticking to this principle will also help your brain realize that it is fully satisfied by the food you are consuming at the normal rate of satisfaction. If you have a problem of "stuffing" yourself, stick with this principle. Sounds like I actually want you to enjoy your meals that you prepare for yourself, doesn't it? Well, it's true; I want you to enjoy your food – slowly. Good and healthy food should be our top priority – and our priorities require time.

Principle Three
Before Getting Seconds... Wait! If you are hungry

and want a second helping of that great meal you prepared, simply wait about five or six minutes. Take a couple sips of water and… wait. Allowing yourself to wait a few minutes will help you realize that you are probably not that hungry. Perhaps you are just "eating just to eat."

Waiting for only five minutes will help reduce your portion size and overall intake of foods! This may be difficult at first, but after three or four days you will get over it and the results will start compounding.

Principle Four
Increase the Field of Your Palate. In Canada and U.S. we are focused on salty and sweet tastes – think of potato chips and mild salsa, or fries and ketchup. Yet, if we expanded our palates to include the other tastes such as bitter, astringent or pungent tastes we would feel more satisfied.

Bitter tastes include green vegetables, astringent foods like apples, pears, or lentils. Pungent foods could be very spices foods. If you have a well balance diet based on a balance of your palate – than you will be able to satisfy your body's need for hunger and hence, over eating.

Principal Five
Don't Eat Until Your Stomach is Empty. This seems like a no brainer. But you can imagine how many people eat just to eat something. Some people eat just to have something crunchy or to compliment whatever it is their doing.

Much of what we eat and how we eat are based on ques. At 12 noon, we eat lunch, because that's when we get our breaks. At 6pm we eat, because that's what we always do. Yet, if your stomach is still working on your previous meal, you should wait a few minutes. Anything less than waiting will expand your stomach and train yourself that even though you are satisfied, you should continue to eat, based on the mental, emotional, or hunger stimulation. With this said, consider having a substantial snack between meals, such as nuts, fruits, or veggies. That along with a tall glass of water will usually help provide the nutrients your body needs (and the fiber) before you next meal.

Your Winning Mind Set & Motivation

Every success story of ours is first written in our mind. In fact, nothing truly meaningful just "spontaneously" happens. Whether we realize it or not, the achievements we have made, all were made possible by determination. It's in our mind that the challenge and victory awaits us.

So, now that we have brainstormed, now we have figured out our goals and their bench marks, the work doesn't end there. Preparing and motiving your mind will help you feed your nourish your goals. Just like a healthy diet of fresh, diverse and nutritious foods, we also need to feed our motivation with diverse elements to maintain

Find Good Reasons to Stay Motivated

Break down your end goal into daily goals and tasks. Resistance training, Cardio and Nutrition. If you're having a day where you're feeling less motivated to stay on track, think about why you have set the goal in the first place and remember that every day you consistently follow your mini goals the closer you get to your final goal.

Some good reasons to keep yourself motivated include: Improving your health, improving your confidence, having more energy and sleeping better. When you reach your goals you get a feeling of accomplishment, you'll be able to walk away feeling great about finding the motivation and courage to stay on track. Every task you complete brings you closer to the ultimate goal, and acknowledging this always feels good.

Your positive attitude matters when it comes to your motivation! Sounds a bit cliché but it's absolutely true. Focus on your positive achievements and not the negatives. All people have some things they are not happy with. Concentrate on the things or people who empower your progress. Stay positive and enthusiastic about your journey and the results you are going to make happen. Remember, that attitude is everything!

Realize that different people may have completely opposite feelings towards the same task: some will hate it, others will love it. Working out and eating right sounds rather boring to many of us. Yet many others love the idea! They like exercising not only because they recognize the good reasons behind it, but also because it's fun! Try listening to music that motivates you and that excites you. In addition, stay clothes to friends that are the same "wave length" and share your vision for what you want to achieve with your body.

Most tasks have a great potential of being enjoyable, and so looking for ways to have fun while working out is definitely a good habit to acquire. Ignore or discount any negative influences or responses to your efforts. Put on your blinders and ear plugs to block out these negative people. Always only take counsel with people who have succeeded in your area before. You must persist!

Time to Take a Different Approach

It's okay to think out of the box. There's always more than one way to accomplish a goal. If a certain approach doesn't work for you, find another one, and keep trying until you find the one which will both keep you motivated and get you the desired results. Some people think that trying a different approach means giving up.

The power of focus is great, but you should be focusing on your goal, and not limiting your options by focusing on just one way to accomplish it. If you work better with competition, make a deal with a friend or family member to compete for the goal! Train yourself to finish what you start by refusing to quit until you are done. Cultivate the habit of determination and persistence.

How to Support your Will Power

Will power is the concept of being able to control our urges, whatever they may be. It is the notion of self-discipline in the face of temptation.

If we don't exercise our sense of will power or self-discipline than eventually we will likely to succumb to our urges. Take for example, "will power vs. cigarette smoking." Will power on its own might not have a chance. In fact, left to fend for itself, our will power has a difficult challenge to stand up to our bad habits. Don't feel bad about yourself as most people have a difficult time breaking bad habits – or really any habits at all!

To strengthen your "will power" or self-discipline, consider a multi-front approach at supporting your decision (whatever that decision is). The first consideration is to remove yourself from that which is tempting you. For example, if you are trying to stop drinking, the last place you should be is happy hour! Sure, you can drink a virgin Margarita, but sooner or later you will cave in. The temptation of surrounding yourself with that which you are trying to avoid is a disaster waiting to happen.

Find a healthy substitution for your habits. When you quit, avoid, or reduce something in your life, consider a healthy alternative to fill its place. For example, if you are trying to quit drinking soda consider carrying a bottle of water with you at all times. (8)

Provide Incentives For Your Success

Reward yourself frequently and at every turn. When you are trying to break a habit and alter your routine for the better, consider an aggressive campaign for rewarding yourself. As long as it contributes to your overall success and it does not compromise your health or your goals in other areas of your life, then do it. It's okay to think out of the box too. The truth is that our brains respond very well to reward at its most basic level.

Rewarding our behavior to institute a healthy lifestyle can be done in a variety of ways – and at the same time. There are plenty of "right ways" to do this! For example, consider a monetary or cash reward system when you have a full day without reverting back to your habit. Spoil yourself in other ways like getting a massage at the end of the week if you follow through with your intention.

Rewarding yourself for a job well done is essential. Make it a habit to work for something. You don't necessarily need to reward yourself using food! There has been some research that food is a powerful primary motivator, which is often used to change and structure behavior in humans – specifically children. What happens however is that children grow up! And when they do something positive, they have already learned to reward themselves with food – and it's often not broccoli! This often impacts our relationship with food, more often in a negative way. This leads to "emotional" eating habits, which we want to cleanse ourselves from!

We have to teach ourselves to reward ourselves with "non-food" items. Set rewards that will push you forward with your "overall" objective. Don't play the "Two-steps-forward, one-step-back" game with yourself!

Take a look Around: Your Environment

We sometimes may not realize this but our environment and who we socialize with often tend to impact our success. If we live a chaotic, unstable, and unfocused life, it would be very challenging to expect any real level of success at anything we do, including enjoying success at achieving better health. Certainly the environments that we put ourselves in tend to influence us both positively and negatively.

My question is: does your environment promote the kind of healthy change you need for ultimate fitness? Is your environment willing to adapt to your change in diet?

The good news is that we can make changes that positively impact our environment. The tough part is "making that break" from whatever elements in our environment that may be holding us back from allowing us to reach our full potential. This "break" is often more difficult that we would like to admit. Let me explain further.

Who We Socialize with is Important

Where you spend your time and who you spend your time with is also essential to this whole process. Consider doing everything in your power to make it more difficult to return back to your habit by making it an inconvenience. On the other hand make your "good habits" easier to reach or obtain.

Who we also hang out with is important as well. Take a look around. Are you being negatively influenced by your friends? The truth is that "breaking" out of your mold includes some changes to the people who influence your life. Change is often a scary thing to someone. For people who surround you, it might make them feel uncomfortable. It might make them feel threatened. Often times, the closest people to you can threaten and hinder your development.

When you change core habits about your life – the way you eat, move towards an active lifestyle, and change what you buy or how you spend your time – all will force people to fill that void in their own life. People often don't like this inconvenience and will react in a number of different ways. Sometimes people might passively resist your changes. Other times, they might be a little more blatantly resistant and discourage your efforts, or even sabotage your goals.

When you begin to change things in your life, it is inherent that you are "taking control" of your life. This essential seizing of control for your ultimate benefits can be very scary and threatening to others. In addition, "they" might not always find that your change is in their best interest. After all, they've gotten used to you and your lifestyle. And it has fit quite well into their lifestyle too. It is not uncommon to find a bit of passive-aggressive resistance or explicit sabotage. It is always helpful to be aware of this.

It is also helpful to find positive people who aren't quite involved in your life to socialize with when it comes to working out and achieving the results you want. For example, a professional trainer or running club members might be a good place to start. When you are trying to break away from the past lifestyle you will soon discover that it's harder than it seems because of the social relationships and molds that have solidified over time.

Let me be clear, I am not telling you to break up with your significant other or stop being friends with your best friend! I am however recommending that you do an honest assessment of the environment and the people who you socialize with in relationship to your goal of weight loss, better health, and ultimately improved lifestyle. **You have to ask yourself and truthfully answer**: Is the environment conducive to your success? Are your friendships – your social support network – conducive to helping you get where you want to be?

Breaking your old lifestyle mold may require you to break up old social groups or friends that have served only to keep you in that rut. A fresh start with small changes always generates great momentum.

Buy In from Those Around You

As you can imagine, changing your lifestyle can have an effect on others. We might not realize that for us to have long term success at creating the healthy lifestyle we want, we need to have those important people – who influence our habits – buy into this new change. We might not be able to split apart from everyone around us, but there are a few things that we can do.

Sometimes, a "heart to heart" conversation is warranted with a spouse, with parents, friends, children, or roommates. Imagine years of buying certain foods like junk food for dinner every week – and then suddenly coming home with a bunch of healthy veggies and announcing to everyone they are going to have eggplant and steamed cauliflower for dinner. This may be bewildering to people around you, especially those who are close to you, like family members.

A "sudden change" may not be taken seriously by those in your "support" network. If your actions threatened their lifestyle, than resistance from those around you may appear to be eminent.

Before making the change, consider talking the changes over your upcoming changes with those who will be most affected by it. But before you have this discussion it's also better to have your own vision and plan in order. You'd be surprised just how many people will not be as supportive as you think. Having your own vision and goals pre-established is essential to come off confident and assured.

In addition, before going out and buying all new workout clothes, healthy foods, etc., consider opening up to those around by first stating how important you think it is to get your fitness and level of health to a better place. Tell them that you want them to help you, support you, and encourage you. Sometimes, people just need to be told what it is that you need from them. Give them the option of joining you, but tell them that you would understand if they didn't want to make any changes. Resolve how the upcoming changes would affect your relationship with them. How will this change how your husband or child eats? How will this effect working lunches or shopping responsibilities with roommates?

Those around you can serve as your biggest supporters and they can also be the biggest roadblock to your ultimate fitness success. It's important that you at least attempt "buy in" and hope to establish your new lifestyle choices with support. Be prepared for anything in return. Be prepared for a little bit resistance. Have your responses ready. Remember this is all about you - about your long term health and about your feelings about yourself. Just how good of a mother, father, or friend will you be if your live life in constant suffering, struggle, and depression? On the other hand, how much better will your relationships be when you are finally at a better place? Will you be happier?

Your Lifestyle Matters

Your lifestyle is made up of the hundreds of habits, both good and bad, and which ultimately determine the life course that you are on. Your state of health, love, happiness, career, etc. all rest on the lifestyle that you - and you alone – determine for yourself. Your habits are created over time by many, many small decisions that are made every single day.

Decisions at home, work, or anywhere in between can shape our habits.

Interestingly, people say or wish they could have the "lifestyle" of someone who is rich or who "has it all" without looking at the habits or what it took to get there. (Grant it, the person who has it all could have inherited everything he owns, but we are talking about the self-made person here!).

Similarly, people may wish they could have the body or "physical build" of someone who has sacrificed and worked on their body's physique and health for many years, without realizing all the healthy habits and hours of training it took to get there. Most often than not, it takes work, sacrifice, and a repositioning of priorities to have a body that looks great.

The point is that when we think about what we want, we generally look at the bigger "lifestyle" picture, without actually looking at the habits that ultimately had to be executed to get there. It takes sacrifice. Anything meaningful takes meaningful time to accomplish.

It's not too hard to imagine that if you have a poor and unhealthy lifestyle you will pack on the calories and in time, develop even more stress, and crave sugary, fatty comfort foods that will, again pack your mid-section with calories. A poor, unhealthy lifestyle creates a snow ball effect.

Remember, success breeds success. Likewise, stress breeds more stress. Unhealthy habits breeds in more unhealthy habits. It's an endless cycle that you need to get a hold of right away.

Simply taking a step back and recognizes that the more stress you have the more stress you will develop over time. Reducing Stress and being better at increasing your time management skills will help you break the cycle.

Why do we eat when we are stressed?

When we are stressed or frightened, our body goes into a protective survival mode – both are pretty much along the same category. In our evolutionary development, humans eat as much as possible when they experience stress or fright for two very basic reasons:

1. The first is to consume enough calories in case the danger or stress causing the event prevents us from eating in the near future. The reaction stores fat as a deposit for future times of danger or inability to hunt or gather for food.

2. Food, especially those with a high sugar and fat content, release chemicals in our body – an endorphin type response which make us feel good. When we are stressed, our body craves for both those reasons.

3. The chemical reaction going on in our bodies and sending signals to our brain can actually be pretty addictive. The feeling is a quick release of stress – if only a temporary solution until we are able to remove ourselves from the threat – is often calmed by the foods we eat.

We're not different from humans thousands of years ago. The problem that our lives are in constant state of stress, danger, and threats is no different from our ancestors, we just have access to very high-calorie rich foods with additives that make it easier for us to gain weight. In addition, there is no need to scour the plains for food.

It is clear, more than ever, that we have manufactured our way to obesity. Our body is constantly craving food and the temporary food highs as a way to protect itself from today's not-so-special anxieties.

The stress locks in your fat and makes it more difficult for you to lose. Large snack and beverage companies know this – they make great tasting, sugary foods that are sold as "healthy" and addictive. They profit and we get fatter.

We have become addicted to highly process low-nutrient rich carbohydrates and need to be free from them. That is why we have created a plan that weans you off these carbs – it is a total plan to develop an attitude and new approach at life, proper and specific workouts to attack your abdominals, as well as your nutrition.

If we take steps to reduce our stress and the need for us to consume more comfort foods, we do three things:

- **We consume less empty calories**
- **We unlock our body's mechanism to let go of our stored fat**
- **We become healthier and able to enjoy life much more**

Stress Factors that Impact our Health & Fitness:

In our modern day lives there are plenty of stress causing stimuli: traffic, noise, deadlines, bills, high expectations, family relationships, and greater uncertainty about pretty much everything. Anything that knocks us off our game, anything that causes a negative physiological change, causes stress.

Undoubtedly, a lot of weight gain can be attributed to stress. So, while it is good to understand that stress creates tons of "weak points" in our will power, we shouldn't resort going toe-to-toe with our desire to eat junk food. The first thing we should do is try to reduce our levels of stress.

Life changing stress factors which are prominent:

- **Death or illness of a loved one**
- **Divorce or relationship break-up**
- **Job loss or job insecurity**

These are just the top three! Other daily pressures of monthly bills, our rent or mortgage due dates, car breaking down, a personal illness, or particular worry about a family member, not having enough time to do the things we want, all settles down in your mind and deep into your stomach – and can have devastating effects on your health and fitness. You worry late at night, so we have a glass of wine with some food. We are rushed to work, so we eat a mayonnaise filled sandwich on the way to our next meeting. We feel that we don't have time to exercise, go to the gym or "take a walk" because we have "more important things to do."

All these serves to multiply the stresses we have. Rather, we need to develop a new way of thinking, a new method of understanding where our stress comes from, taking steps to remove the stress before they settle in and attach themselves to us. We need to chip away at the old stress factors that have calcified and solidified themselves to us.

Let me share with you what may change the way you look at stress, food, your health, your weight gain/loss:

The food we eat while stressed is stored and metabolized differently than the food we eat when we are relaxed. When you are stressed your body is producing various chemicals that signal that these nutrients you are taking in need to be stored and packed away. This of course makes losing weight that is gained during these conditions even that much more difficult!

This is why it is so important to deal with life's common stressors. Sure exercise, eating healthy, and making good choices are important to living well, but we will never reach "total wellness" unless we address those things that are stressing us out.

Ways to Tackle Stress

I have identified a few things that help me reduce the stress in my life that I think are worthy of mention and consideration here. By consistently addressing the stress in our lives, we can do more for our health, weight loss than you can imagine.

Sleep:
This can be the hardest thing for people because we often chip away at our sleeping schedule to get things done. Stress might even cause insomnia which in turn leads to other conditions such as fatigue. Studies show that having proper sleep hygiene is essential for weight loss, a slowing of the aging process, muscle building, elevated moods, and clarity. Getting enough sleep and rest habitually needs to be a priority.

Simplify:

Simplify everything: relationships, partnerships, work schedules, daily schedule, weekly schedules, and your role at work – simplify. Simplify. Simplify. We tend to often complicate our lives – all the time! We are sending texting messages, emailing our friends, all while checking the weather online – as we are driving! We cannot only see the danger in this, but do you see the information overload we are all experiencing. All this keeps us distracted and simultaneously increases our stress levels - and decreases our productivity.

Instead let's try to turn off the television, read your email only twice a day, don't be a slave to your cell phone, and prioritize your jobs. Your top priority of work should be attacked from 8am to 11am – every day.

Plan Ahead:

Life will always create stressors for us. We know this. We know that something always will happen that is unexpected. We will have setbacks. We will have dark days from time to time. So, shouldn't we plan for this?

I knew a man who planned for his bad days by stocking up on tons of alcohol. A wrong choice for me, but in his own way he planned for his negative days. I am asking you now: can we plan for bad days in a positive way? For example, can we plan to have a particular yoga or Pilates workout, or meditation, or prayer for times that are tough? Can we nurture healthy friendships that can cultivate positive energy when we need it the most?

Acceptance of Things We Cannot Change

Sometimes we get so stubborn. We want to control everything. We want to change what can't be changed. We want to control what we can't control. It stresses us out. It fills us with anxiety. It causes us to overeat and be non-responsible. What if we just accept things that we can't change?

While this may be easier said than done, learning to accept the things the way they are and keep moving forward is an excellent strategy to stay on track. When we get riled up, we usually trip ourselves back into a healthy routine. By staying focused on what matters, we can insure that we are doing all that we can to stay within reach of our goals.

Prioritize and Re-examine Everyday:
I discussed a little earlier that creating priorities can be very impactful for us. Yet "priorities" by themselves can be rather futile, without any action behind them. What I have found that breaking our priorities down into steps can be very helpful. A priority of "eating healthy" for example, can be broken down a series of action points and measures of time.

So, let's take eating healthy as one example: *It is my priority to eat healthier this month.*

Okay great. It is now your priority to "eat" healthier this month. It's a good goal. But to add some "teeth" to our goal let us include a few action steps that we can measure. Consider the following:

Your action steps may include:

1. Making a meal plan
2. Shopping for the right foods

3. Making more time to cook
4. Reducing "unhealthy" drinks and snacks

Keep it simple. You don't want to overwhelm yourself. Focus on the few that you know you can work on when you give them a little attention by prioritizing them. Do you see how we are first creating a general goal and the creating specific action points? Do you see how I am not telling you to go cold turkey and make a promise to the diet gods that "you will never have another piece of chocolate" in your life? I don't do that because, if you remember when you were a teenager, rules were meant to be broken!

Give yourself room to fail and time to adjust. Allow yourself the flexibility to change in a methodic, slow, and uncompromising way.

In addition, our lives can take up a lot of time with a lot of "stuff." You'd be amazed about how much stuff we put into our lives simply because we don't want to do the one or two things that we should really be prioritizing. Remember get rid of your clutter! You should prioritize your job into what is essential to what is not. Categorize your jobs into: what must be done now, by the end of the day, and within the week.

Make a list and follow it by the following order of importance:

- **By the end of day**
- **By the end of the week**
- **By the end of the Month**
- **60 days**
- **90 days**

These points aren't set in stone. Whatever works for you will do fine, but you have to do something. You have to create a measurable goal. Why? Because you can manage or control, what you can't measure. Once you are able to measure it, you'll be in control of it. Sounds a bit abstract, but it's true.

Prioritizing might also mean having the ability to say "No" at times. The word, No, can be very effective at helping reach our goals too. Likewise, the word "Yes" can be the surest way to get further and further away from the goals we set for ourselves.

We don't often like to hurt others, so we say yes, when we really can't afford the time, effort, energy, or money, we often go along because it is the path of least resistance. Believe me, I know. I have been there myself. But our ability to successfully prioritize the meaningful things in our lives means that we need to have the ability to say "No" when it matters the most.

Try it this week. Say "No" to someone or something that happens to be cluttering up your life and you day to day routine. Say no to wasted energy and time on unnecessary drama or gossip, or conflict. Living a healthy life also includes removing and separating ourselves from "time and energy leeches." You can be nice and gentle about it. Saving no can be a very liberating experience.

Although as awkward as it may seem at first, saying No will begin to free you up for all the important things that you need to get to. It makes room for your priorities to breath and action to take place.

Here's something you probably already know. Humans seek pleasure and avoid pain. Diets that deprive us of feeling "satisfied" will lead to other consequences, such as binge eating, hormonal imbalance, moodiness, fatigue.

Sleep & Hunger – A New Perspective

Our relationship with hunger and sleep is often dysfunctional. The more dysfunction we have with these two essential parts of our lives, the changes are that we will struggle with our weight.

Hunger isn't a nuisance. Just like being "sleepy" isn't a nuisance. It's a survival signal that our body is trying to tell us something important. As I stated before that I am true believer in the "Law of Attraction." One of the premises of the "law of attraction" is that we shouldn't focus on what we don't want. We should "fight" against something we don't want, but instead fight for something that we do want.

Too much of a good thing? With an abundance of foods and sugary snacks our society has seen our

123

weight increase rapidly. A mix of marketing of what "ideal beauty" all manufactured by big business, we have struggled with dieting staving off hunger. This has impacted women tremendously and recently started to have a negative effect on men too.

In fact, our western culture has been losing the hunger wars – that is, that we have spent the last 50 years coming up with strategies to "fight" off our hunger. Diet pills, supplements, food items like rice cakes, teas, and a number of other different products have been added to the arsenal to combat the feelings of hunger. Nearly every single diet out there has done one of two things, added to the hysteria that you "hunger" is a sign of weakness or that you aren't eating right or it is something that you should never feel.

Let me ask you something right here – what would happen if you lost your ability to feel the sensation of hunger? How better or worse off will you be? Certainly, many people who are ill or have medical disorders are unable to feel hunger. Unfortunately for many of them, their ability to survive long-term without any help usually isn't promising. Let me be clear, our body's ability to produce a hunger sensation is essential to our survival and well-being. If we stop fighting it, we will all be better off!

The fact is that we need our feelings of hunger. Hunger is a physiological necessity, just like the feeling of being cold, hot, frightened, or sleepy. Just like any other sensation our body tries to communicate with us. Hunger is an intimate feeling that we should not try to "numb" with pills, supplements or teas. Now, certainly today's big food industries have added plenty of chemicals (additives) that some research has been shown to manipulate our feelings of hunger. Refined sugar addiction is certainly one that many of us struggle with.

The perspective of being "at war" with our natural hunger has distorted our relationship with food and our bodies. The first thing that is implied is that we shouldn't trust our bodies!

It's so amazing for me to run across some very intelligent and well-intentioned people who spend much time meditating and practicing breathing exercises to connect with their bodies, and then do abnormal things to fight off their hunger!

I often think that our feelings of being "hungry" and being "sleepy" can be compared to each other fairly regularly. Being sleepy is a natural feeling (as is hunger) but our relationship with sleep, although isn't as bad as our relationship with hunger – we often do everything in our power to prevent the feeling. Sooner or later, no matter how many cups of coffee or caffeinated drinks you have, no matter what strategies you employ, your body will demand sleep.

As you probably know from firsthand experience, that sleep deprivation can cause a number of problems if we don't get enough of it, your ability to be productive will decrease sharply. But we all know that no matter what we do to prevent sleep, sooner or later we will have to get it.

Interestingly, stress, a lack of sleep, and poor nutrition all increases are cravings for carbohydrates and fat. But what is really happening? Stress, anxiety, worry, all increase our levels of cortisol, which tells are body to maintain its grip on existing fat and slow down your metabolism! If you are stressed for a long period of time, this will obviously impact our testosterone and estrogen production, our serotonin levels, and of course alters our mood.

Finally, what are benefits of being fit and healthy?

Being fit and healthy doesn't solve all of life's problems. You still have to pay your bills, you still have to work, and you will still have to cope with a lot of life's ups and downs. Rather, being fit and healthy allows you to be better prepared – physically, mentally, and emotionally for whatever life throws at you. Being fit and healthy certainly creates an advantage for dealing with life's ups and downs.

Here are the added benefits:

- **Looking great**
- **Feeling your best**
- **Able to do more physical activities**
- **Able to feel confident about yourself**
- **Provides a great outlet for everyday stress and anxiety**
- **Avoid many illness and diseases caused by sedentary lifestyles**

By just making a few changes in our diets by increasing our fiber we could reduce a number of various cancers by a third! (You are what you eat). Additionally poor diet leads to more miscarriages and infertility issues. A diet high in sugar can cause poor level of concentration lead to conditions like diabetes and obesity.

Summing Up:

Certainly making small and impactful decisions every day can really make a big difference over the span of a week, two weeks, a month, and a lifetime. Realizing our full potential for a high quality life based on health and fitness is with reach. Working on our attitude, motivation, perspective, and our decisions takes real attention, but once we do, we are certainly walking down the path towards our goal. No doubt prioritizing, developing a vision and a set of goals, supported by a specific plan to reach those goals in a manner that can be measured is essential for our success. But the fun is just getting started. With this in mind, let's start focusing on our nutrition.

Go to
www.totalwellnessbook.com
For FREE tools!

Turn this great book into a wellness support system by downloading templates, documents, recipes and other great tools!

Chapter 2: Nutrition

"Let food be thy medicine and medicine be thy food" - Hippocrates

I have learned so much about dieting during my career as a trainer and as a fitness competitor. One important thing that I learned is that our nutrition and our eating habits are often based on an emotional component.

Certainly, beyond the actual food we are eating lays a deeply rooted emotional aspect of our health, fitness, and dieting. It's not so hard to consider how foods play a role in our lives. We remember our childhood kitchen filled with Mom's cooking, Grandma's cookies, seasoned holiday foods, family picnics, and barbeques. The act of eating together as a family, among friends, and colleagues is a social action that is very bonding. It is very commonly all based on some emotions.

Understanding and acknowledging this very common occurrence of most of this is empowering. Learning to separate our emotions from our eating can unlock much of our dependence on food for comfort, security, and intimacy.

You want to be able to eat a healthy balanced diet without having your life revolve around it. It is one thing if you are getting paid to be a spokesperson for a supplement company, then yes it is your full time job to prepare 6-8 tiny meals a day consisting of fish/chicken and vegetables. But usually this isn't the case.

I can't stress the importance of balance and moderation. I myself have the most ridiculous sweet tooth. I've never been one to crave fast food but I am never too full for desert! Most people will say that if you have to "cheat" with food to do it early on in the day when you are sure to burn it off through your daily activities, work, etc. or right after a workout when your metabolism is at its highest. I find though that emotionally it easier to have your cheat meal late in the day instead of early when you are likely to keep eating bad the rest of the day.

The more sugar you eat the more you will be craving it the rest of the day the more likely you will keep cheating all the way until bedtime anyways. This is just one example of how emotion and will power play a big part in planning out your nutrition.

Food is an enjoyable part of our lives. I truly believe that we shouldn't outlaw good taste or enjoyment. Our body evolved to make healthy foods enjoyable. Developing a realistic plan for our diet regimen is important but it doesn't have to leave us with a feeling that we are missing out.

Mix up your diet during the week. Choose at least one new organic fresh food to eat. Lentils and other legumes are excellent sources of fiber and protein. Fish is an excellent source of protein and fatty acids. Always include nuts and seeds in your diets. Nuts and seeds can provide protein, vitamins and minerals, and a number of different enzymes. Many nuts contain Vitamin C, B, calcium, magnesium, zinc, and iron. Try and limit yourself to only a couple of tablespoons of nuts and seeds per day.

If you are addicted to sugar – consider berries or fruit as substitutes.

Diversify your meals. Have fun with food. Discover great things to make that are healthy for you and your family. Food is simply one of the best things in life – allow yourself the freedom to thoroughly enjoy healthy food.

Add some spice – spicy meals tend to satisfy the palate in a way that distracts your body from craving more sugar.

Add some color – real, natural color! By adding color to your plate you will encourage a variety of vitamins, minerals, and enzymes that are beneficial to your health. Additionally, you can provide some diversity to your palate, stamp out sugar cravings, and train your body to crave new tastes.

The Importance of Nutrition

Your health and fitness begin and end with nutrition. And it should be the foundation of reaching your goals. Certainly no matter how hard we train or exercise, we will not be able reach our goals unless we find a way to increase our healthy eating.

Every single day our bodies are bombarded by stress, pollution, and anxiety. In addition, a good majority of us go through our day dehydrated and lacking enough in-take of vitamins and minerals we need. That is not to say that we aren't getting our share of calories – we certainly are! But calorie intake and essential intake of vitamins, minerals, protein, and the "right" kind of fat is often lacking.

A few days on a very poor diet, we basically are functioning on a much depleted body. How can we expect to look and feel our best feeding ourselves refined sugar, fats, oils, and walking around dehydrated? It's nearly impossible! A couple of days of poor diet and our moods will begin to change, our metabolism changes, our skin changes.

How to Shop For Food

Without a doubt, your health and fitness begins at the grocery store. No matter what you do, you simply cannot out-train your diet. The choices we make at what we buy at the store each week, will often determine much of our success and failure at the gym.

With all of life's challenges, who has time to cook up a great meal? Or go through the hassle of even preparing for one? The fact is that if you want to change our body composition and increase our fitness then we need to focus on our buying habits.

Taking control of your grocery spending habits is liberating. I know it might not seem that way at first, but when you take control of your weekly meal planning, you actually can mentally, emotionally, and physically free yourself. (9)

Consider the following when it comes to our purchasing habits:

Mental liberation: Do you know how much we think about food? "Um, what am I going to have for dinner?" or "I don't know what I want, let's just order out." The truth is that we dedicate a lot of time during the week just thinking about food but without doing any planning. When we are mentally drained and don't know what decision to make, chances are we are going to settle on the "path of least" resistance. And while the path is paved with good intentions, we usually succumb to eating something that isn't healthy – because it's easy, convenient, satisfies our pleasure zones, and it has been a habit for years!

Emotional liberation: The truth is that many of us eat food and the type of food due to emotional reasons. By planning your meals ahead you simply nix out the emotional aspect of our eating habits to during the week. If you have difficulty eating healthy during particularly stressful times in your life, meal planning is especially important.

Physical Liberation: If we shop and plan for groceries on a whim, we often find ourselves going to the store 2-4 times a week. When you consider the commute time, shopping time, waiting in line, and putting groceries away, this can take away an extra 4-5 hours a week or 20-25 hours a month! Why not spend that time exercising, sleeping, or simply doing whatever it is that you love!

Of course, the other important aspect to planning ahead is the inherent savings. Study after study shows that planning ahead when it comes to shopping for food saves time and money. Over the course of months or years, the savings could be significant.

It is no secret that the best way to shop around most grocery stores around America and Canada is to shop around the perimeter of the stores. It is within the belly of most stores is where much of the processed, high-calorie, and sugary processed foods exist. Instead, start in your produce section first. Choosing organic is my preference because of the reduced exposure to pesticides and other chemicals. Stock up colorful foods and mix up your selection. For example, try sweet potatoes, beets, and jalapenos to your meals.

For your carbohydrates consider whole grains such as quinoa, bulgur, and millet. When choosing your cereals, consider oatmeal instead of the packaged granola or other "healthy" cereals which are often packed with sugar or other artificial sweeteners.

Making Bad Choices Difficult to Make

Most of the time, we know when we are making bad choices or healthy choices. A high percentage of this time we make the wrong choices because it's the path of least resistance. Yet, if we turn the tables around and make the "healthy" choices easy to make, and the "bad" choices hard to follow through, then we decrease the gap that lies between us and our success.

Balancing Protein, Carbs, & Fats

Increasing your protein intake and reducing your carbs and fat are essential, especially when we are talking about a typical North American diet. Protein is essential increasing our lean muscle mass, but it also an important energy provider as our bodies convert the majority of our protein intake into glucose. (10)

In general we want to avoid things foods that "spike" our blood sugar levels. Where carbs and sweets tend to do this, protein consumed moderately doesn't have a dramatic effect. This in turn doesn't leave us with the "crash and burn" feeling.

Fat is packed with calories, which the body converts only 10% to glucose for energy. Fat intake also slows down our digestion and though it doesn't generally spike our blood sugar levels, it keeps our levels higher. Now we know there are "good fats" and "bad fats." Fats derived from olive oil, canola, avocado, and nuts are healthy mono-unsaturated fats are healthy because they actually lower or "bad" cholesterol levels. On the other hand, saturated and trans-fats found from fats coming from animals and dairy products are those we want to avoid. (11)

Together these three nutrients - fat, carbohydrates, proteins — all which contain calories that your body uses for energy. Here's how to balance these nutrients in a healthy diet.

Our Water Intake

Most likely, our bodies need more water. If we are working out, stressed out, or changing our diets and habits, we need to drink more water. Unfortunately, by the tie you are thirsty your body is most likely already dehydrated.

No doubt that being hydrated is essential to good health. Without proper hydrations our organs can function properly, our blood and brain are effected are muscles fatigue, our toxins can't flushed, our digestive system suffers, wrinkles on our skin appear, and we just feel horrible. Drinking is essential throughout the day, but your body is particularly dehydrated when you wake up in the morning. Instead of grabbing that coffee, first get a full glass of water!

You've probably heard that drinking eight full glasses of water every day is the standard. The real truth is that your appropriate water consumption varies on a few factors including how active you are and where in the country you live.

Water is essential to your body at it is the primary chemical compound in your body making u 60% of your body's weight. Not only does water help our organs function properly, but it also helps flush out toxins as well as carry the necessary nutrients or bodies need.

Sports Drinks and Beverages

If you spent any time at the gym recently or if you have been out for a hike, you will be surrounded by people who are consuming sugar water. Expensive sports drinks and caffeinated drinks have been a success of beverage companies and their marketers. The truth is that these sports drinks don't hydrate your body better than say, water and a piece of fruit, which contains natural sugars and water. In fact, all they do is pack on the calories and make it harder for you to lose weight.

Question: But what about all the athletes that you see on television drinking sugary drinks? Well, those professional athletes may be drinking your favorite colored sports drink, but they are also burning thousands of calories during a game.

In addition, they probably burn through so many calories during the week that they can afford to have drink or two! Even if you buy the "zero-calorie" beverages, your still packing a lot of synthetic chemicals in your body that stimulates hunger sensations, with no real benefit except make your wallet lighter. If you are exercising or trying to detox your body naturally, don't substitute your water with sugar drinks – no matter how good the marketing is. It doesn't make sense and it's not worth the money!

A doctor and expert in nutrition from Yale University can back me up on this. All this "marketing is based on the gimmick that somehow this extra load of sugar and calories will turn you into an athlete," he told

America's National Public Radio. These marketers have handily convinced that people should drink this sugar water before, and after workouts too! (12)

Stay away from sports beverages, fancy sports gels, etc. The truth is that they are full of refined sugar, which actually dehydrate the body and cause you to overheat. Why would anyone pay for that?

Eating Good Fats

Fats are not evil. In fact, you cannot get the body you want without "good" or healthy fats. Fats are vital to the great body composition that you want because fat is used to create the lipid layer of cells that serve as an integral part of the production of muscle building hormones, which includes testosterone. Since higher testosterone levels are associated with better body composition, included healthy dietary fat is essential.

Yet, confusing the two main types of fat intake can be disastrous to our health. The key is to eliminate "trans fats" and "hydrogenated fats" from our diets, because they destroy the "insulin" receptors in our cells. In turn this destroys our metabolism, which helps us to burn off energy efficiently. In addition, Trans and hydrogenated fats increase our LDL (bad) cholesterol levels which are responsible for clogging up our arteries. It's easy to find Trans fats in hydrogenated foods, which we want to avoid as much as possible.

Omega-3 fatty acids on the other hand are healthy fats. In fact, they often counter the effects of unhealthy fat. The best Omega-3 is found in fish oil, which contains DHA and EPA. Diets high Omega-6 fats, which come from corn, soy, peanut, and vegetable oils has been associated with inflammation and increase the risk for some cancers. While Omega-6 fats are unavoidable, aim for a diet that his near equal ratio between Omega-3 and Omega-6. (13)

Coffee/Caffeine

If you are like most people in North America and Europe, you're first drink in the morning isn't water or juice, but coffee. In fact, nearly 50% of all people in the North America have coffee just after they stumble out of bed.

The studies on coffee on its health benefits and negative effects go back and forth as industries and other substitutes try to influence the behavior of consumers. However, what I am concerned about is that many people incorrectly substitute a proper diet, which includes coffee instead of real and nutritious energy.

There have been studies linking coffee to the difficulty in absorbing vital nutrients, vitamins and minerals. However, I tend to believe that coffee is a numbing agent. It is a legal and widely used drug that tricks us into thinking that our body is feeling fine or "awake" when it really needs is adequate sleep and rest. (14) Do you remember what I said about our relationship with food and sleep? Coffee or caffeinated beverages have an impact on our relationship with adequate rest.

Other health concerns to drinking too much coffee/caffeine include:

- Potentially higher cholesterol levels
- Loss of fluid in your body
- Insomnia
- Anxiety symptoms
- Depleted calcium & Iron levels in women

The unfortunate reality is that our awareness of coffee is often molded by a profitable coffee industry. The U.S. alone imports over $7 billion in coffee every year. Multinational companies spend millions of dollars on coffee ad campaigns that persuade you to buy coffee. They convince you that this drink is indeed safe and healthful for your consumption, reducing your risk of diabetes and other illnesses, even when they don't have enough solid evidence to prove this. (15)

With all that being said, is coffee horrible for you? It won't kill you but, there are simply other alternatives that are healthier for you to consider.

Why You Should Switch to a Healthy Non-Caffeinated Alternative

This has been an issue that has long been hidden from the public and I believe it's about time that someone in the health industry speak up and reveal the real score behind coffee drinking. I firmly believe that you should try your best to break your coffee habit and turn to a coffee alternative, without the dangerous ingredients and without the health risks, as soon as you can. In reality, the caffeine in coffee does not create real energy or alleviate tiredness. It is only provides a strong stimulant that provides a sudden, temporary jolt to your system, hence the feeling of alertness but it's side effects can be too much of a cost to take on.

The Dairy Problem

We have been sold a myth: That milk does a body good. Like coffee, another large mainstream staple, is the dairy industry. Today's dairy industry doesn't provide the same products that our grandmothers enjoyed several generations ago. The milk we drink isn't the milk that our grandparents enjoyed.

Unfortunately, the route that transforms "healthy milk" products into allergens and carcinogens begins with feeding methods that big dairy farmers impose on their cows in the name of profits.

Here are the basics, in order to get more production from cows, they are fed a diet of hormones and injections, which is said to enlarge their pituitary glands, among other side effects, so that they can produce much more milk than your traditional "everyday" cow that our grandmas used to drink from. The result is that these cows need antibiotics to keep them healthy because their hormonal levels have derailed their immune systems. (16) If you think that those chemicals, hormones, and antibiotics are being passed through into our bodies, than you find yourself on the side of reason.

The second ridiculous thing comes next. The cow's milk is quickly pasteurized so that all valuable enzymes that would be healthy for us are then proficiently destroyed. Literally dozens of other essential nutrients and enzymes are destroyed in the pasteurization process. Without them, milk is very difficult to digest.

In addition, the butterfat of commercial milk is homogenized, which quickly turns it rancid. Even worse, when butterfat is removed altogether, it makes for a great marketing product due to its lower calorie level. We call this "skim" milk. Skim milk has been mislabeled and marketed as healthy, but we're really drinking empty calories because without the fat, our bodies can process the remaining nutrients.

Ah, so what happens next? Of course, synthetic Vitamin D is added to your milk. I am always weary of foods that need to be fortified, because that means somewhere along the process it got the nutrients stamped out of it. The words "fortified" or "enriched" should always draw up red flags.

Other Factors Regarding Milk

Some research point to milk and refined sugar as the two of the largest contributors to food-induced ill health. That may seem like a totally harsh thing to say, but when one examines the evidence, this is a reasonable conclusion. The recent approval by the FDA of the use of Bovine Growth Hormone by dairy farmers to increase their milk production only worsens the situation. That means dairy farmers have been given the green light to max out their cows production by pretty much any means legally necessary, which means pumping their cows with hormones and antibiotics. We don't have to be an agricultural expert to understand that the hormones and chemicals cows are injected directly affect the nature of their milk. Not sure about you, but I don't want to be at the end of a glass of BGH packed milk.

But shy the concern over BGH? Some research has shown that BGH causes a spike in an insulin-like growth factors or IGF-1 in the milk of treated cows. This IGF-1 does survive milk pasteurization and human intestinal digestion. It can be directly absorbed into the human bloodstream, particularly in infants. Why does this matter? Good question, some research has indicated that it is highly likely that IGF-1 promotes the transformation of human breast cells to cancerous form. We think of milk as being healthy, regardless of how it's produced. So, as you can imagine, milk (and cheese) producers don't have to sell you on the nutrition of milk because we already assume it is.

While certainly there are benefits to milk, consider the added issues we need to think about that occur along the production chain to get to our kitchens every week. Getting more out your money and nutrient investment, when we're talking cows here, might be great for dairy farmers, but is it healthy for us? You decide.

Detoxing Your Body

We have all heard of detoxing diets or programs, right? You might have actually tried a few. Unfortunately, the temporary benefits simply don't outweigh the negative effects. But "detoxing" our body might sound good. It might seem intuitively correct to get rid of all the toxins in our body, right?

But too often these detox diets or programs are extreme, calorie and food restricted plans based on the 'concept' of removing harmful toxins from our bodies that result from preservatives, food additives, insecticides or our bodies own waste products. In theory it sounds convincing, but it's really not. Nevertheless, let's take a quick look.

How do "detox and cleanse" programs work?

These programs are said to work by limiting or completely eliminating foods from your regular diet for a designated period of time, usually a day or up to a week (or other specified time) depending on the type of program. Because these detox programs sound convincing and are profitable for their creators, there are plenty of cleanses and diets out there. Basically they all follow a very low calorie regimen, with small portions of fruits and vegetables and water. Some supplementation with herbs, vitamins, and powders to cleanse the colon is also given. The supplements can be very expensive and the effects have always been called into question.

Do Detox Regimens Generate Weight Loss?

The answer is usually yes. However, it's no secret that the weight loss is only temporary. (17) The weight you actually lose is simply "water weight" which often returns when your resume your regular diet. The question is that should we detox our bodies? I would say no. The fact is that our bodies have the ability to do this function on its own pretty effectively. If we want to detox our bodies, then a complete reduction or even elimination of alcohol and smoking will allow your liver to do its job.

Additionally, the effects of a "detox" might be harmful. Some studies suggest that when we diet with "juice" or detox our bodies in some other way that appears to be extreme, it responds quickly to the sugar intake and we get a spike of insulin production. As we use that sugar our sugar levels drop, which can leave us feeling fatigue. In other words we can experience a sugar crash. Since you have eaten much, your body goes to the liver and muscles for energy.

After the first day, you can be fatigued. Next your body goes for its long term energy sources, fat cells and your actual muscle. After a couple of days, your body becomes concerned and enters a "semi-starvation" period. Because your brain also needs amino acids, which it is not getting by your detox, feelings for depression or "brain" fog set in. Since you are using your muscles for energy, the break down creates ammonia and uric acid, which are unleashed into your blood stream. This is a huge toxic cleanup job that your body is actually doing. Now your liver and kidneys are working overtime to detox the effects of the detox. This obviously isn't good. Well into your first week, you are prone to diarrhea, your small intestines are not happy because there isn't food to digest and you have lost plenty of muscle mass. (18)

And this is only the beginning. What happens when you return to your regular diet? Well, your body just experienced near starvation which triggers the "famine effect." We've talked about this earlier. This affect basically tells the body that food is scarce and you need to not let go of any of the calories that you eat in the future, ultimately slowing your metabolism and making it harder and harder for you to actually lose weight! In addition, to regain the loss in muscle will impact your metabolism rate.

The truth is that when you make the effort to keep yourself hydrated, choose healthier meals, exercise daily, de-stress, and make healthier lifestyle choices, your body is able to naturally detox by itself.

How to Stop Sugar Addiction

Consuming sugar is the fastest way to increase your fat supply around your midsection. It is also one of the most addicting chemical compounds in the world, so I know that it's especially tough to beat sugar addiction.

Consider one study from France that was discussed at the yearly meeting of the Society for Neuroscience in 2007, which emphatically showed that when mice where given a choice between sugar water and cocaine, nearly 95% of them chose the sugar water. "Even rats addicted to cocaine, switched to sweetened water when given the choice. In other words, intense sweetness was more rewarding to the brain than cocaine" (19)

While writing about sugar addiction isn't the scope of this book, there are a few things that you can do to break free from this powerful addiction.

1. **Choose better substitutes. For example, less processed foods are packed with sugar. Highly processed foods essential burn away the taste, so sugar and other additives are put in its place.**
2. **Don't start the day with sugar - donuts, pancakes, and sweetened muffins.**
3. **If you are tired and fatigued, don't alleviate your feelings with sugar. Take a nap, rest, and get better sleep.**
4. **Keep high sugar sweet out of your home at whatever cost. Don't bring home a large pack of donuts that the folks at work "would just throw away!"**

Remember that sugar is in many seemingly non-sugary foods we eat, like ketchup, salad dressings, granola cereals, etc. Reexamine your sugar intake by

Hormones and Our Health

There are 24 different hormones that affect the appetite. Our hormonal levels effect the way we eat, sleep, feel, metabolize food, and everything in between.

Hormones play a key role in our "weight loss" or "weight gain." Manual Villacorta, in his book, *Eating Free,* focuses on one of them in particular that has a dramatic effect on weight gain or loss. The hormone is called *ghrelin*. Do you remember earlier, when I discussed the concept of a "famine response," which occurs when we severely restrict our diet? It is one of the biggest negative side-effect of crazy dieting.

Ghrelin is a powerful hormone that is secreted into our stomachs when we are hungry. It may trigger the physiological response to hunger. When we deny our hunger sensations, more ghrelin is quickly produced and goes on to spark more hunger sensations, this time in our brain. Suddenly, our mind and our body are demanding us to eat. (20)

In a tip of the hat to will power, we ignore these signals. We think we are doing the "right thing" and feeling great about ourselves. But while we are feeling good that we are conquering our body with our sense of will power, what is old *Mr. Ghrelin* up to? Hmm. Well, it's now signaling to your metabolism to slow down – way down. It tells your body to stop burning fat! How does this impact our will to maintain course on our dieting?

Ghrelin is basically saying, "Hold up! Hold up! We're not going to be fed anytime soon, so don't you dare let go of those love handles!"

Diets that merely focus on a blanket sense of "will power" are really just preventing us from losing the weight we want. Now, don't get me wrong, I think there is a place for will power. But we have to use it for the "right" things – not to hamper our ability to reach our goals!

Interestingly, avoiding carbs or not eating enough of them and your ghrelin jumps up. So, what does this tell us? Well, we certainly need to have a mixture of protein and complex carbohydrates to keep ghrelin down to normal levels while we work out. We do this by eating substantive nutrients every few hours. A healthy snack or meal every 3 to 3.5 hours can keep ghrelin at bay or at least normal levels. (21)

In addition, this also tells us that losing weight by skipping out on meals doesn't too well for most of us in the long run. You don't want to trigger a famine response in your body. Fasting for anything other than religious, cultural, or other similar circumstances, should be discouraged in my opinion. The small and insignificant short term gain, don't cover the medium and long term costs to our body and mind.

The Portions We Eat Always Needs to Be a Consideration For Us

Fortunately from hard work of activists and progressive owners, many restaurants can provide labeling information. I believe we should use those labels to help us to make healthier decisions for ourselves but also avoid certain chemicals, additives, and preservatives. But I am also pretty realistic. I don't count calories every day. I don't count calories all too often in fact. I just don't think it's realistic to sustain over a lifetime. Unless you are a pre-diabetic or you are focused on a specific dietary issue, counting calories just isn't that important.

Rather, what I do focus on is portion sizes and a mixture of dietary nutrients in every meal. While you may have seen and have your own opinions about the movie, "*Super Size Me,*" by Morgan Spurlock, the fact of the matter is that most people are eating way too many "calories" by consuming whopping sizes of highly caloric, oil-rich, sugar-packed meals with very little nutritional value. The average restaurant plate serves way too much food, usually in the form of simple, highly processed carbohydrates and simple starches.

Fats:

The fact is that although we like to demonize fats, we need fat to survive. Fats allow us to absorb a number of vital nutrients, help break down other fats, and help us to synthesize our hormonal levels.

There are three types of common fat:

- **Saturated fats** – often found in meat and dairy pro, like cream, butter, and milk.
- **Unsaturated fats** – often found in fish like salmon, fruits like avocado, and olive oil.
- **Trans fats** – often found in packaged, baked items, like muffins, and fried food. These are the fats we should try to avoid, if not completely eliminate from our bodies.

I believe that we should avoid, a nearly all costs, to consume Trans fats. However, unsaturated fats are essential and should be eaten in moderation. You simply can't think to substitute your trans fats for unsaturated fats and still call it a day! Remember, consuming everything in moderation helps you stay on track.

Restaurant Eating:

Like most people I think going out with friends and family to restaurants can be a fun social event. But believe it or not, restaurants can be effective places at piling on the extra weight. A couple of nights out for dinner, a few lunches per week with co-workers, a brunch on the weekends, and we are talking thousands of extra calories per week that we don't need. To put it simply, food that is made out of your house is simply out of your control. For us to get and stay in control of our weight, our fitness, and our health, we need to stay in control our food source nearly all 100% of the time.

Now, I'm all for going out and having fun. I have few favorite restaurants that I enjoy, but many of our favorite restaurants cook with tons of butter, sugar, salt, fats, and rich creams, sauces, that are packed with everything we try to avoid. In addition, the portion sizes are often huge, packing enough calories to sustain a grown adult man for a couple of days.

Some Strategies When You Eat Out

There will be times when you eat out. Some of us eat out quite often. There is no question that foods from restaurants often contain more fat and trans-fat, sodium, non-organic fillers, heavy creams and oils, than the food you eat at home. However, I understand that we all need to eat out from time to time.

Here are a few strategies to help you:

- **Study the Menu – always look for meals that have the most healthy nutrients**
- **Keep your food separate – a mix foods combined together often has the most oils, fats, etc.**
- **If you are ordering vegetables, ask the waiting staff to have them steamed.**
- **Always ask for sauces and dressings on the side**
- **When you eat out, cut your portions in half**
- **Drink water only**
- **Choose fish is a healthy choice when dining out. Ordering seafood such as**

salmon and tuna adds Omega-3 fatty acids to your diet

- Avoid fried and cheese products
- Avoid high sodium foods that are easy to eliminate like pickles, salted pork, etc.
- Ask your waiter is you are not sure how food is prepared
- Avoid gravy, creams, or butter sauces
- Ask your veggies to be steamed instead of sautéed
- Choose meals that are broiled, baked, or grilled
- Pass on the fries, onion rings, or fried zucchini
- Skip on the desert or share it with friends
- Cut the portion in half, and take a box home

Keep in mind that this is not about creating more rules for you to follow, but rather it's about retaining some of your control in restaurants.

Most of the time, you simply don't have control over what is put into your meal. Why would you allow that? By asking and making some better decisions, you can take better control of what you eat every day. If you would like to eat some of the items that are on the menu, like a variety of sauces, desert, etc. consider making them yourself at home. This way you know exactly what is going into your body.

Age Factors

Over the course of my years in training, I have seen quite a few excellent examples of men and women in the forties, fifties and even seventies who are in excellent shape. There is no question that working out, eating right, focusing on our goals, allow us to look our best, and help us to move towards the direction of our goals with determination and clarity.

While research has indicated that our metabolism, muscle mass, and optimal hormonal levels drop slightly each decade after we hit adulthood, I have met amazingly fit and well-muscled men in their 60's and 70's. In addition, I have met great looking and motivate women who work out in their 70's and 80's! Interestingly, all of these individuals have a couple of things in common: an amazing attitude and a zest for life! The power of our attitude doesn't often get the attention it deserves, but it is still important.

Whether, you are 27 or 87 we can make healthy decisions every day that can have an immediate and positive impact on our life.

A Life Long Goal of Health

The fact is that life isn't a sprint. It's a *series* of sprints and a *series* of marathons all at the same time, with hopefully some great periods of rest in between. I'm not sure how it all started, but someone convinced us that we can eat horribly for years and wipe it away within 21 days or 30 days, or whatever the trend is. These fleeting and often harmful diets don't serve to help us, as much as it does encroaches on our ability to truly tackle our health and fitness by cluttering up our mind and thoughts. It also keeps us in this no-win cycle of poor health, erratic dieting, and long term weight gain.

What if I break my health routine?

Okay, so you have decided to move forward with a new healthier you. But as it sometimes happen, we break apart from our new healthy routine and eat a whole pizza by ourselves. Or we go to a friend's birthday party and have too many alcoholic drinks. The list can go on and on. But one thing is for sure, the next day we might feel really guilty and thinking, "What have I done?"

Many people get discouraged and decide to go back to your old lifestyle. Something (perhaps your guilt or feelings that you used to have come back) and tell you that you don't deserve to have the body or the health that you want.

But stop, right there! First, just because you had an "off-night" or slightly strayed from your new healthy routine, doesn't mean that you have blown it completely. You're body doesn't work that way. Instead of compiling daily averages, consider that your body works in "weekly averages." While calories and the types of foods that consumed – and the amount of exercise done – is averaged throughout the week. While you might have had a bad night consider that it still doesn't affect your "weekly average." Therefore, don't throw in the towel simply because you had a "bad" day or someone got off your diet. Instead, simply go for a walk, plan out your meals for the rest of the week, and continue.

Integrating your Nutrition and Diet with Your Exercise

I recommend high intensity work outs, longer fat-burning workouts, and strength training. Combining these three umbrella workouts can help you burn fat, increase strength, change your body composition, and help you feel great – all while complementing your eating habits. These three will generally lead to about the same metabolic rate change. In other words, when we're talking fat loss, they will all generally be the same. And yet they serve very different purposes that are beneficial to us. Certainly, these different types of workouts offer slightly advantages over the other in regards to strength, endurance, and speed.

Let's take a look this issue a little further:

For better health, this is what you should look for in labels.

Total Carbohydrates: This is a catch all total for grams of fiber, sugar, and "other" carbs, which add up to the total.

Dietary Fiber: This is the part that is not digestible.

Sugars: This will tell you the total amount of carbohydrates from the sugar in the food and it will often combine added sugar and natural sugar.

The Basics of a Gluten-Free Diet and How it Can Help Us

A gluten-free diet is a diet that excludes the protein, gluten, which is can be found in a variety of grains such as barley, rye, and wheat, and others. A "gluten-free" diet is generally used to treat celiac disease, which can cause inflammation in the small intestines of people who have the condition. While you might not have celiac, you still might have slight allergic reactions to gluten, which often goes un-diagnosed. For example, you might have an upset stomach, headaches, or feel fatigued, or you may have a skin reaction. There are a number of different seemingly unrelated reactions that may occur without knowledge.

Eating a gluten-free diet assists those people with celiac disease control their signs and symptoms and prevent any complications.

As you might imagine, following a gluten-free diet may be frustrating. But with time, patience and a bit of culinary creativity, you'll find there are many foods that you already eat that are gluten-free and you will find substitutes for gluten-containing foods that you can enjoy.

Labeling for gluten free products vary among countries. Australian standards reserve the "gluten free" label for foods with less than five parts per million of gluten, as this is the smallest amount currently detectable in food. (22)

Many healthy and delicious foods are naturally gluten-free:

- Beans, seeds, nuts
- Fresh eggs
- Fresh meats, fish and poultry
- Fruits and vegetables
- Most dairy products

In addition, many grains and starches can be part of a gluten-free diet:

- Buckwheat
- Corn and cornmeal
- Flax
- Hominy (corn)
- Millet
- Quinoa
- Rice
- Soy

Avoid all food and drinks containing:

- Barley (This includes malt, or malt flavoring and malt vinegar are usually made from barley)
- Rye
- Wheat

By avoiding these foods I have been able to feel better, keep those stubborn pounds off me and generally control those afternoon "crashes" that we are all too familiar with. Too much sugar by common foods like bread, crackers, chips, can lead to wild swings in our sugar levels.

If you have struggled, as I had for many years, to get through the afternoon blues during the week, we may point to our dependence on gluten and the sugars that spike our blood sugar and then it comes crashing down.

More on Gluten Labeling

In general, avoid the following foods unless they're labeled as gluten-free or made with corn, rice, soy or other gluten-free grain:

- Beer
- Breads (sprouted breads are okay)
- Cakes and pies (crust)
- Most Candy
- Cereals
- Cookies and crackers
- Croutons
- French fries
- Sauces
- Imitation meat or seafood
- Pastas
- Salad dressings
- Seasoned rice mixes
- Seasoned snack foods, such as potato and tortilla chips
- Soups and soup bases
- Vegetables in a variety of sauce

I know what you're thinking: "Oh, Taya, this is going to be challenging" Well, to some of you would consider stop eating all of these at once and going cold turkey. While others of you will consider phasing out your foods and learning to replace them with other much healthier options. It is really up to you. There is no one-size-fits-all here and I am not going to tell you what's best for you and your family. You know that this is going to be a personalized diet for you.

Certain grains, such as oats, can be contaminated with wheat during growing and processing stages of production. For this reason, doctors and dietitians generally recommend avoiding oats unless they are specifically labeled gluten-free.

You should also be alert for other products that you eat or that could come in contact with your mouth that may contain gluten.

These include:

- Food additives, such as malt flavoring, modified food starch and others
- Medications and vitamins that use gluten as a binding agent

Watch for cross-contamination

Cross-contamination occurs when gluten-free foods come into contact with foods that contain gluten. It can happen during the manufacturing process, for example, if the same equipment is used to make a variety of products. Some food labels include a "may contain" statement if this is the case. But be aware that this type of statement is voluntary. You still need to check the actual ingredient list. If you're not sure whether a food contains gluten, don't buy it or check with the manufacturer first to ask what it contains.

Risks of Gluten Free Food Consumption

It is important to remember that there is no "magic bullet" when it comes to your health. Certainly eating a gluten free diet may work for you and be advantageous. However, your exercise routine, your lifestyle, and other choices in what you buy are just as important to your health.

Not getting enough vitamins

People who follow a gluten-free diet may have low levels of certain vitamins and nutrients in their diets. Many grains are enriched with vitamins. Avoiding grains with a gluten-free diet may mean eating fewer of these enriched products.

Ask your dietitian to review your diet to see that you're getting enough of these key nutrients:

- Iron
- Calcium
- Fiber
- Thiamin
- Riboflavin
- Niacin
- Folate (Folic Acid)

Not sticking to the gluten-free diet

If you accidentally eat a product that contains gluten, you may experience abdominal pain and diarrhea. Some people experience no signs or symptoms after eating gluten, but this doesn't mean it's not damaging their small intestines. Even trace amounts of gluten in your diet may be damaging, whether or not they cause signs or symptoms.

A protein found in wheat, barley, and rye (and countless food products - like bread and pasta - that contain those grains), gluten gradually damages the intestines of people with celiac disease, preventing the absorption of vitamins and minerals and setting off a slew of related health problems, which can include fatigue and bad skin.

Gluten intolerance of any kind, including celiac disease, is often underdiagnosed (or misdiagnosed) because it manifests itself in many and murky ways that can baffle doctors.

If you suspect your body can't tolerate gluten, the first thing you should do is get tested for celiac disease. If the test comes back negative, try a gluten-free diet for a week to see if you feel better. Cutting out gluten is the most reliable way to determine if you are, in fact, sensitive to the protein, and if you are sensitive, it's the only treatment.

The Gluten Conclusion

There have been tons of books and articles written on gluten. I've simply given you a brief intro to something you may consider doing to improve how you feel and reduce the weight we continue to battle with. While cutting out gluten from your diet may be healthy, simply cutting out gluten doesn't make you healthier. Remember, this is simply one a part of a process of being healthy, which includes a healthier lifestyle. Interestingly, gluten and this issue helps to remind me that what we do eat is important and how we react to it in a sensible way that makes sense for each one of us as individuals is even more important.

Eliminate All Processed Foods

When we think about it our grandparents and their parents didn't depend on processed, packaged foods. Fresh fruits and vegetables were the norm. While we are living longer today, the percentage of us have cancer is skyrocketing.

Eliminating processed, packaged foods is essential to our overall health. We just have to make this a priority – not just to look better, but to feel better. To put it

plainly, processed foods are all-around bad news –
more sugars, more trans fats, more chemicals, more
preservatives, more GMO ingredients, and less
nutritional value.

And while eliminating all processed foods from your
diet should be one of your goals, we can also be
tough. So, here is what I recommend. Start by adding
more fresh fruits, vegetables, and lean meats into
your diet. The more you introduce the less "space" for
other things, such as packaged goods. In fact, this is
something that I suggest to people that are interested
in dieting. By simply "crowding" out the foods we want
to avoid, we can feel satisfied and steadily create
healthy habits in eating.

Packages goods lack nutrition, generally contain
chemicals, dyes, and artificial additives, and the
macronutrients have been modified or are denatured,
which means they aren't metabolized in the same way
as if they were in the unprocessed state. The
chemicals and additives in processed foods increase
your toxic load. All of these chemicals must be
metabolized and removed from the body, which can

overload the body's natural detoxification system. For the same reason you need to eat organic as much as possible, but eating organic processed foods does not provide a complete solution either.

To be sure the best fat loss results will come from removing processed foods completely from the diet. I have seen many people look and feel better with just doing this.

Many people don't realize that even foods such as cereal, bread, and energy bars that say "made with whole-grains" or "great source of protein and fiber" on the package are still highly processed and should be avoided.

Over the last several years, I have looked a variety of diets. While I am not an advocate of "dieting" I do believe that certain "diets" have some nuggets of great information that is scientifically-based and proven to help. Incorporating the benefits into a cohesive and comprehensive diet that you can sustain for life and weaving a healthy diet regimen into your new lifestyle is certainly important.

One of the dieting regimens which has made an impact on my life and which I incorporate into my personal daily diet, comes from the Paleo Diet. To my knowledge and from my experience, this diet is probably one of the best diet regimens I have come across in my years as a trainer. (23)

To be sure the Paleo Diet follows along similar types of foods every single person on the planet had eaten since before the Agricultural revolution. A diet that included fresh foods (fruits, vegetables, lean meats, and seafood) all which are high in the beneficial nutrients, such as soluble fiber, antioxidant vitamins, phytochemicals, omega-3 and monounsaturated fats, and low-glycemic carbohydrates.

The Paleo Diet, in my opinion, promotes good health as it eliminates refined sugars and grains, saturated and trans fats, salt, high-glycemic carbohydrates, and processed foods. All of these frequently lead to weight gain, cardiovascular disease, diabetes, and numerous other health problems.

The Paleo Diet encourages dieters to replace dairy and grain products with fresh fruits and vegetables, which foods that are more nutritious than whole grains or dairy products. It is diet humans have been specifically adapted to. This program of eating was not designed by diet doctors, faddists, or nutritionists, but rather by Mother Nature's wisdom acting through evolution and natural selection.

While not for everyone, consider how you can incorporate such wholesome nutrition into your daily diet. I know that while training to stay in shape, build muscle, the Paleo Diet doesn't take away from necessary nutrients my body needs. The Paleo Diet is based upon extensive scientific research examining the types and quantities of foods our hunter-gatherer ancestors ate. This nutritional plan is totally unlike those irresponsible, low-carbohydrate, and high-fat, fad diets that allow unlimited consumption of artery-clogging cheeses, bacon, butter, and fatty meats. Rather, the foundation of The Paleo Diet is based on eating lean meat, seafood, and unlimited consumption of fresh fruits and veggies, which is the diet our ancestors used. (24)

No our modern life today and life back then were of course considerably different, however, if you strip all of today's modern conveniences and looked at a healthy adult who had to be physically active and have the use of all of his or her faculties to live productively, the Paleo Diet can be beneficial. Here is a diet that not only sustained human life but allowed it to thrive in the harshest conditions.

The Paleo Diet does a good job in my opinion of addressing any criticism that might be found in your typical diet. For example, it is true that hunter-gatherers studied during modern times did not have as great an average lifespan as those values found in today's modern industrial nations. However, most deaths in hunter-gatherer societies were often related to the accidents and trauma of a life spent living outdoors without modern medical care, as opposed to the chronic degenerative diseases that afflict modern societies.

When taking a look at most hunter-gatherer populations today, about 10-20% of the population is

60 years of age or older. These elderly people have been shown to be generally free of the signs and symptoms of chronic disease (obesity, high blood pressure, high cholesterol levels) that universally afflict the elderly in western societies. When these people adopt western diets, their health declines and they begin to exhibit signs and symptoms of "diseases of civilization."

The carbohydrates (unlimited fruits and veggies) in The Paleo Diet are of a low-glycemic index, meaning that they cause slow and limited rises in your blood sugar and insulin levels.

Further the Paleo Diet is consistent with how I feel about drinking cow's milk. There's no nutritional grain requirement for humanity or any other primate that can't be met by other animal and plant foods. Similarly, humans have no nutritional requirement for the milk of another mammalian species throughout our lives.

As a species, we can get along fine without either of those food groups. The novel concept promulgated by the USDA and other governmental agencies and public institutions is that these food groups are required by all humans for optimal nutrition. In fact, as we have pointed out in the scientific literature a number of times, grains and dairy are nutritional lightweights when it comes to the 13 micronutrients (vitamins and minerals) most lacking in the U.S. diet. Fresh vegetables, seafood, lean meat and fresh fruit are all more nutrient dense than are whole grains cereals and whole milk.

Paleo Diet encourages dieters to replace dairy and grain products with fresh fruits and vegetables — foods that are more nutritious than whole grains or dairy products.

Organic and Genetically Modified Food

Unfortunately, in the name of profit and efficiency the food the majority of us eat are compromised. Shot up with hormones, vitamins, antibiotics, and other drugs to create fatter meat, more productive cows, may have more of a significant impact on us than many of us realize. I believe that more current and future studies will shed like on how dangerous genetically modified are effecting our health, the health generations yet unborn, and the environmentally negative impact it causes. Fortunately, there are alternatives, which may cost the average person more in comparison to the cheaper GMO foods available.

The organic movement in North America has inched its way through appealing to more and more people despite the giant and powerful food industry's domination over the food market. Consumers today have responded by demanding natural and organically and locally-farmed food, which is minimally processed. While slow to start, the organic and natural sales have grown to include 12% of the market.

Read the Labels

Despite the downturn in the America, European, and world economy over the last several years, consumers have increased their demand for higher priced foods. Consumers, more conscious than ever are now beginning to understand that organic and natural products may be healthier and friendly to the environment, more humane for animals and equitable for farmers.

While processed foods are known to be "cheaper" the fact is that these foods have plenty of hidden costs in government subsidies, environmental damage, and health care costs.

Because many companies know that there is a drive for organic and naturally (minimally processed) foods, they have slightly altered their marketing tactics, branding, and promotion of their products. Companies are scrambling to change their labels without doing much to the original products. This means that we need to be vigilant about the foods we eat. We should always read the labels!

Buying Organic Is Essential But Shop Smart

But what does "Certified Organic" or "USDA Organic" mean? We hear "organic" all the time, and today assume it to be good. But what does it really mean? And should we stay vigilant about the things we eat? For starters, the label of "organic" means these products are certified to be about 95-100% organic. Certified Organic means the farmer or producer has undergone a regular inspection of its farm, facilities, ingredients, and practices by an independent Third Party certifier, accredited by the USDA National Organic Program. However, consider that small family farmers may be just as good. The certification process can be expensive and simply obtaining the labeling process each year might be too high of a barrier for many smaller family farms.

What about "Natural" label products?

Unfortunately, "natural," in the overwhelming majority of cases is meaningless, even though most consumers do not fully understand this. Natural, in other words, means conventional, with a green veneer. Many "natural products" are often produced using pesticides, chemical fertilizer, hormones, and genetic engineering.

Natural or conventional products-whether produce, dairy, or canned or frozen goods are typically produced on large industrial farms or in processing plants that are highly polluting, chemical-intensive and energy-intensive. "Natural," "all-natural," and "sustainable," products in most cases are neither backed up by rules and regulations, nor a third party offering organic or natural certification. (25)

Behavioral Relationship with Food

To really lose the weight we want, feel great, and be happy, alert, and motivated over a long period of time, we will need to change our engrained relationship with food. In addition, we also need to be aware of the sophisticated marketing tactics used by big food business who hire seasoned marketing/advertising experts who study our habits, our fears, our wants, needs, desires, and understand our "trigger" mechanisms (wanting to be skinny, environmentally-minded, and healthy) to sell us their empty calories.

Our relationship with food is founded on our self-image, our idea of "will power", among other things. Don't you find it ironic that the very thing that provides us our nutrition, our ability to live, and deliver it wonderfully the pleasure of taste, smell, texture – has all been cast out as evil. "Food" is not the enemy.

Food is certainly one of life's most wonderful pleasures that we should all enjoy every single day. From the smells all the way to the taste, food not only sustains us physically and mentally, but also provides a way for us to indulge our senses. This pleasure point in our lives should be celebrated, not demonized, as it has been for the last half-century.

Certainly in our North American culture, our food and our consumption of it is generally done in the setting that is almost always rushed. Certainly, a culture that invented, lives, and depends on "fast food" we are now beginning to pay the price, in our rates of obesity, chronic diseases, environmental degradation, supporting huge agricultural business that make it tough for small and local farmers to be sustainable.

You knew it was coming: A few Do's and Don'ts

Here are a few do's and don'ts that I usually incorporate into my lifestyle. Consider each one and how it might impact your life and health.

Stop Drinking Carbonated Drinks (Even diet drinks): Research has indicated that diet drinks lead nutritional deficiencies due to the inability to absorb nutrients and lowers your metabolism. Get more sleep. "I can survive on 4 hours a night," one of my clients said. The fact is that people vary in their sleep needs but most people need 7-9 hours of sleep. Sleep hygiene affects your metabolism rate. In addition, being sleep deprived makes you want to pick up that can of power drinks...or that donut in the morning.

Here's a quick list:

- **Eat your breakfast! Not having a breakfast often lowers your metabolism rates.**
- **Drink water between bites**
- **Schedule more time for your meals**
- **Slow down while eating**
- **Chew more**

- Shrink your dinner plate – literally
- Don't buy anything with an "–ose" at the end. Fructose or dextrose are just synonyms for sugar.

Eating Organic is essential:

In his book, **The Weight loss Cure** *"They" Don't Want You To Know About*, author Kevin Trudeau argues that food manufactures are creating foods that are designed to increase our hunger. "Food manufacturers are making food with the sole purpose of creating a physical chemical addition to the foods. I have personally been in the chemists' labs where the directives are to create food that increase hunger, lower metabolism, get a person physical addicted to the food (like a drug), and make people fatter," Trudeau writes. (26)

He goes on to say, "This is why food is ripened with poisonous gas, injected with chemical preservatives and flavoring agents, eradiated, pasteurized, bathed in poisonous chlorine baths, injected with antibiotics, growth hormones, and other deadly drugs.

Learning from your Personal assessment

It's easy to write stuff down and then plop in a drawer somewhere never to be found or looked at again. Writing down everything that you eat isn't always easy. So, if you take the time to write everything down, you should also take a few minutes to go over your weekly averages.

After about a week of writing down everything down that you have been eating, get a highlighter pen and circle the obvious choices.

The process of writing everything down and examining the assessment at the end of the week can help you develop a greater sense of awareness about what you eat, when you eat, and how much you eat. In addition, we are able to focus on our diversity (or non-diverse) meals. Are we eating too much fat? Are we having too little protein? Are we consuming too much sugar? If you have faithfully have been writing, then your list will provide you quite a bit of insightful data.

I can't stress the importance of our food being the cornerstone of our health. The food we eat fuels are body. But it also *heals* our body too. In fact, our bodies are in constant state of repair. Every single cell needs the nutrients that we provide for it daily. In turn, whether or not our cells get their needed nutrition, influences our moods, our attitudes, our endurance, our ability to feel good about ourselves.

You probably already know that our health depends on our nutrition, but let me illustrate this point a little further.

Let's say that we go out to our local fast food restaurant and get a hamburger, fries, and a soft drink totaling 18,000 calories, mostly consisting of fat, sodium, and sugar. In addition to having very little nutritional value the meal sets triggers you to feel exceptionally good for about 45 minutes to an hour. Then you start to feel the crash. Additionally, this "crash" caused by spiking and spiraling insulin levels also wreaks havoc on your moods – so you begin to feel horrible about your body, you begin to feel depressed, and your sense of empowerment goes out the window. Sometimes you might even feel like giving up on your healthy eating plan altogether because you feel that you have to be a slave to sugar and fat.

While I want to encourage you never to give up – your health and the path to fitness is sustained by daily and even hourly decisions. Okay, so you went out and had a "bad" meal? Get over it and start again. The thing about eating is that you do it several times a day – every day. So, it's never too late to start again.

Here is my advice for having a bad meal.

Don't Stress: Don't panic or create extra stress for yourself. We all from time to time make poor eating choices. The trick is to not get bogged down with your overall goal. Keep your eye clearly focuses on your goal.

Walk: Go out and take a walk as soon as you can. This will help immediately burn off the calories you just consumed.

Water: It is essential to drink lots of water – this will help flush out toxins and keep your organs healthy.

Fiber: Eat an apple – this will help you from your upcoming "crash" and provide necessary fiber for your colon.

Plan Ahead: Instead of being down on yourself. Consider planning your next healthy meal. This will often re-invigorate you to eating healthy.

These five simple points of action can go a long way to helping your stay on course. They will help you to not get slogged down in an emotional state of helplessness that many of us feel after eating a meal or two that are not the healthy. Remember, you might have occasional "slip ups" but your success is your ability to maintain your positive attitude and focus for the long run. Don't let one or two meals or events trip up your goals.

Go to
www.totalwellnessbook.com
For FREE tools!

Turn this great book into a wellness support system by downloading templates, documents, recipes and other great tools!

Chapter 3: Fat Loss/Diet

Be Smart, Avoid the Fat Trap

When starting your exercise program it is vital to avoid what is being called "The Fat Trap" with proven strategies that will make you feel better and help you lose the weight you want. You want to eat a high-protein diet, strength train, and eliminate cravings that might sabotage your plan. You also want to supplement your plan to help give your metabolism the boost it needs.

An intriguing and recent study written in the *New England Journal of Medicine* sheds a bit of light the long term physiological influences of severe calorie restriction on hormones that influence metabolism. This means severe dieting. The article pointed to what not to do if you want to have a lean body composition. Specifically, it stated that we should restrict calories, and certainly not to an extreme level. But we do want to modify our macronutrient makeup to avoid turning your body into a hormone-induced hunger machine, and be sure to perform regular physical activity. (27)

Hormones that promotes metabolism, such as Leptin is often reduced by a strict calorie restrictive diet and a hormone; in addition another hormone called Ghrelin, which actually promotes fat storage is significantly elevated in the body. When combined, this endocrine profile will set anyone up for difficult struggles with weight management and make it virtually impossible to maintain an even weight, let alone lose more weight.

Don't Count Calories

According to research a much more effective, affordable and beneficial solution for better health and body composition, is an approach that doesn't restrict or count calories, includes a physical activity program, and helps individuals eliminate cravings.

There's abundant evidence that a high-protein, low-carb diet will help with weight loss, and calorie restriction is not necessary. There's even evidence that it's not necessary or even a good idea to eat low fat as long as the fat you eat is the right kind—"good" fats in the form of omega-3s. Also, it's essential that you optimally balance your fat intake with an equal ratio of omega-3 to omega-6 fats, while eliminating all Trans fats.

To get rid of cravings for high-carb and "bad" fat-filled foods, the best bet is to eliminate them from the diet. Research shows cravings will decline if you make the effort to not eat selected foods that trip you up. Supplementation is also a better solution than severe calorie restriction because if you get your omega-3 fats dialed in, take carnitine, and ensure you're not deficient in the basic nutrients (zinc, magnesium, vitamin D), you'll feel better, be more motivated, and have a much improved metabolism.

Surprisingly, the researchers in the "fat trap" study don't mention a need for getting people active and strong. Strength training is absolutely crucial for fat loss and body comp because by gaining strength, you'll build muscle, burn fat, and elevate anabolic hormones such as testosterone and growth hormone.

In addition, there's also evidence that intense training will raise leptin, lower ghrelin, and blunt hunger. Plus, training and physical activity will improve insulin sensitivity, glucose uptake, and fight chronic inflammation!

For best body composition results, the answer isn't complicated, elusive, or very difficult. Eat high protein and low carbohydrate meals. Strength train is important. Make sure you get the essential nutrients and consider adding other supplements that aid metabolism. Eliminate foods that you crave but trip you up (Remember, think about the big picture here!) Make it a lifestyle and you'll feel better.

Remember, Stick to Portion Sizes

We talked about this briefly, but sticking to moderate consumption during multiple meal times is important and deserves another mention. Having several meals a day and snacks in between works great for many people. Instead of gorging on food a couple of times a day, providing moderate-sized portions is a way to spread out the calories needed throughout the day.

Carbs - Reducing Body Fat

The fact is that we need carbohydrates in our bodies. And while the debate ranges back and forth about the effects of carbs on our bodies. Collectively, we have both feared and embraced. So, which is it? Should we fear them or use them to our advantage – which is getting the type of body we want?

The evidence and research is becoming clear that carbohydrates are double edged sword that can be used for good and bad. The negative effects are determined by which ones we choose. The good news is that it's easy to tell the difference between the two types (good and bad). (28)

Good & Bad Carbs

"Good" carbohydrates are packed with fiber. The more fiber they have the better for our digestive system, but these carbs get absorbed slowly into our systems which has means that they don't "spike" our insulin levels. These kinds of carbohydrates include sweet potatoes, black beans, and broccoli.

Those bad carbs such as white bread and white rice tend to spike our insulin levels up. Certainly a total ban on carbohydrates simply doesn't make sense like some popular diets profess. The fact is that complex carbohydrates play a key role in our health, fitness, and hormonal levels, moods, and level of energy.

The National Academies Institute of Medicine recommended that we start focusing on increasing our fresh fruits, vegetables which will increase our intake of fiber in our diet. The NAIM recommended that the average adult get about 45-65% of our calorie intake from complex carbohydrates. This would include about 20-35% from fat, and 10%-35% from protein. Since we are working out, we should lean on the higher end of protein, and the lower end of the fat and carbs. (29)

The only healthy way to get our necessary carbohydrates which are packed with the fiber we need is through plant foods. While we already know the risks of low-fiber diets such as heart disease, digestive problems, we know also know that it can help prevent colon cancer and help with weight control.

It is recommended that men in their 40s and 50s get a higher intake of fiber, which is about 38 grams a day, where women should get about 25 or more grams of fiber. Healthy Fiber derived from plant food has cellulose which humans cannot digest but is helpful to our intestinal track, but it also generally means that nutrients come along with it, such as necessary vitamins and minerals. Because it moves through our system slowly dropping off much needed nutrients, it also makes us feel more satisfied and less hungry throughout the day. More importantly it can help stabilize the spikes in our sugar levels, reducing the risk of getting Type 2 Diabetes.

Avoid White Sugar or Fructose

The Carbs we need to avoid are white (refined) sugars, or added fructose. We simply eat way too much sugar. There's sugar in our ketchup, in our teriyaki sauce, our cereals, our breads, our coffee, and our drinks…our spaghetti sauce. You name it, and it probably has it. If it doesn't come from cane sugar then our sugar sweeteners come from corn syrup, which is found in soda and many, many other products – some of which are label "healthy." The sweeteners can pack on the pounds quickly.

While the USDA recommends that we get no more than 10% of our daily calories from added sugar (which is about ten teaspoons), I say that's till way too much

We need fat. We couldn't survive without it. There are a few types of fat that are essential and play an important role in our health. The first type of fat is needed to protect our organs, our joints, and ensure that our skin is youthful and supple.

Our reserve fat which is what we need for good health is what our body uses for fuel and it is this fat that is burned off when we diet. This fat plays a role in our joints and organs as well. The third, and abnormal or excessive fat is what we really want to lose. They are often located in "problem" areas. This type of fat is only released during severe nutritional times. (30) A better way to release this is slowly, over-time, with attention to diet and exercise.

You've seen the advertisements before. Dietary hunger suppressants. Many of supplements are distant cousins of "speed", which fill you up with caffeine and other chemicals. However, did you know that exercise is one of nature's best and most reliable appetite suppressants? That's right, it's in our nature to suppress appetite when we are doing something physical. When you are "feeling" hungry although mentally you know that you are satisfied, consider going for walk, take out the garbage, mow the lawn, etc. Creating an active lifestyle starts with making small and seemingly mundane choices every day – even every hour.

Taya's Fat Loss Tips

We have all created wonderful goals about losing weight that are for the most part, as vague as they can get. "I need to lose some weight." Or "I want to get back into shape." Sounds good, right? But does it ever happen? Well, it might for a short time that is until we get back to our "normal" routine.

Consider the following Fat Loss Tips:

Add Protein to Our Breakfast

Start off the morning with about 30 grams of protein. This helps jump start the fat burning hormones Starting your day off with an egg may help curb your appetite better than cereal, new research suggests.

In a small study, it took longer for people who ate eggs for breakfast to show signs of hunger than it did for those who had a bowl of ready-to-eat cereal. Scientists suspect that egg protein may be better at making people feel full longer compared to the protein found in wheat

Supplements - Reducing Body Fat

While eating a healthy diet, supplements play a major role in our health. As we have discussed that the best exercising our bodies comes from strength training. In addition to our intense workouts, we also live an active lifestyle that uses up plenty of nutrients that we need. When much of our focus is in strength, weight loss, and body composition we need to understand that our bodies require supplementation of nutrients to keep it going strong. (31)

To be sure, there are no substitutes or "supplements" for a healthy diet and exercise regimen. But ensuring that your body had the right supplements it needs will promote, support, and maximize your efforts. Avoiding vitamin deficiencies, especially while training, is essential. And believe me, even if you are on a great and well-balanced diet, you can burn away plenty of vitamins and minerals quickly.

Supplements can help the body burn the fat you have already deposited. In addition it can lead to a rise in protein synthesis and detoxify our bodies, flushing out the toxins that are produce constantly. Supplements can also support our hormone levels so that we optimally burn fat.

Supplement #1: Probiotics
Probiotics, which are tiny and healthy bacteria found in our intestines, are important to maintaining a

healthy digestive system. Guess what? If you don't have a healthy digestive system then your "healthy" diet will not matter much.

A healthy digestive system maximizes its ability to absorb the needed nutrients, break down proteins, and expel toxins. In addition, the health of your digestive system provides a way for us to get certain essential compounds like Vitamin K. There are some suggestions that probiotics help us lose fat.

These friendly bacteria are essential to our health, but they can be easily outgunned by "unfriendly" bacteria, such as E. Coli. In addition, if we find ourselves taking antibiotics, a class of drugs that is designed to kill bacteria, then we especially need to supplement our diet with probiotics.

Supplement #2: Get Your Omega-3s!
It is true that fat has gotten a bad rap. Too bad because just like fighting fire with fire, we can also fight unwanted fat with fat! That's right! By now you may have heard about the benefits of Omega-3. Omega-3 Vitamins provide anabolic benefits that help

build muscle. Omega-3 supplements are vital because they support your body's efforts right down to the cellular level. Cells in our body contain a double layer of fats, which often determines how well our metabolism works. The need for healthy fat is essential because if it filled with "bad" fat then your cells will not bind well with insulin.

Supplement #3: Magnesium, Zinc, and Vitamin D There is no question that these three supplements help maintain a healthy metabolism. Let's consider each of these individually. Vitamin D helps with the absorption of calcium and in addition dials down the volume of enzymes that cause the body to store fat. Magnesium supports cardiovascular health and overall physical performance by regulating the heart function. In addition, it has been known to reduce to reduce stress. Zinc is a powerful antioxidant and anti-inflammatory. Additionally, Vitamin B Complex can help flush out toxins that we are sure to produce when we are exercising.

Avoiding Common Pit Falls

Over the last year or two, I have personally been trying to limit the amount of sodium in my food and in doing so I began to feel better, less bloated, and had more energy. I highly recommend that you do the same.

For starters, I don't normally cook with salt, which is a great way to limit the amount of sodium you get right off the top! Fortunately, we usually have great natural seasonings without sodium, so I don't have to compromise on the taste of my food!

With the obvious consideration out of the way, here are ten simple ways to reduce your sodium intake:

1. Drink less soda. Diet soda especially has quite a bit of sodium.
2. Eat less fried foods. Though many of us love fried food, which is not that healthy for us to begin with, we often add plenty of salt.

3. Eat less canned soups which often contain tons of sodium.

4. Avoid cured meats, such as bacon.

5. Realize that some "fresh" meats are also injected with sodium. This helps preserve the meat and it also "packs" on some "weight." Since we know that meat is sold by weight, guess who benefits?

6. Limit condiments, such as ketchup and barbeque sauce.

7. Salad dressings often have lots of sodium too!

8. Chocolate bars have plenty of sodium so check the back of the labels and compare!

9. Reduce your intake of butter which often has loads of salt (buy non-salted butter).

10. Baked goods often have sodium. Read the labels on your bread.

Whey Protein:

Whey protein is a high quality protein naturally deriving from milk. Whey protein is a complete protein containing all of the essential amino acids your body needs and is easy to digest. Whey protein is also one of the best sources of branched-chain amino acids (BCAA).

• The amino acid profile of whey protein is almost identical to that of skeletal muscle.

• Provides a high concentration of branched chain amino acids (BCAAs) to maintain and repair lean muscle tissue following exercise and to prevent muscle breakdown.

• Provide BCAAs to help maintain adequate stores of glutamine to limit muscle breakdown and a decline in immune function.

• May increase glutathione levels to help improve body composition (sustain lean muscle), enhance exercise performance and help maintain immune health.

• Helps stimulate muscle protein synthesis after exercise to reduce muscle damage and improve endurance.

• Easily digested, high quality protein to provide additional energy.

• Provide BCAAs to help prevent fatigue during intense, longer duration sports events

• Helps athletes maintain a positive nitrogen balance to minimize muscle breakdown and enhance muscle repair/recovery. (32)

Supplements can be an excellent way to shore up your intake of vital nutrients, especially while you are working out. I have used Shaklee supplements consistently, whether I am in training or not. Why Shaklee? There is clinical documentation available behind every single health claim made by Shaklee about its products. This cannot be said by other nutrition companies who utilize anecdotal information about general perceptions of a nutrient's effectiveness.

Additionally, Shaklee is the ONLY nutritional company that can make the following claims:

It has invested over $250,000,000 in research and development of its products. It has over 100 published studies and abstracts in peer review journals that prove efficacy of its products. Further, over 75 scientists on staff to develop breakthrough products which enhance your well-being. Over 50 patents on unique products that are only available from Shaklee Landmark Study proving

Shaklee supplement users have markedly better health.

No doubt, when you choose Shaklee, you get the best of nature:

All natural ingredients

No artificial flavors

No artificial sweeteners

No hidden fillers

No animal testing

**Go to
www.totalwellnessbook.com
For FREE tools!**

**Turn this great book into a
wellness support system by
downloading templates,
documents, recipes and other
great tools!**

Chapter 4: Diets:

Everyone has a different situation and your diet will have to be unique to you. Everyone has different levels of carb sensitivity, time for preparing, some people are always traveling, some people cook for only themselves and other people have to cook for their whole family.

The bottom line is to eat clean, know how to read a label or if possible stay away from foods with labels all together. If you are going to have "cheat" foods try to make sure they have some nutritional value. Don't starve yourself or restrict calories, eat small portions every couple of hours. The Paleo Diet addresses this and it makes the most sense to me. Here is the definition of that diet:

The Paleo Diet is "centered on commonly available modern foods. The "contemporary" Paleolithic diet consists mainly of fish, grass-fed pasture raised meats, vegetables, fruit, fungi, roots, and nuts, and excludes grains, legumes, dairy products, salt, refined sugar, and processed oils."

So, what I have done personally and which is helped me achieve great results in my life is the following diet regimen. Stop Dieting! Yo-Yo dieting is one of the worse things do to your body.

Consider the following example diets that you may want to consider. While there is no "one size fits all" consider that you may want to rearrange the following example diet plans to best suit your needs.

Athlete Diet Example

Day	1	2	3	4	5	6	7
8:00 am	40 min cardio	Break	40 min cardio	40 min cardio	40 min cardio workout	40 min cardio	Break
9:00 am	1/3 cup oatmeal	4 egg white omelet with veggies	Egg white pancakes	Scrambled eggs, once slice toast	Omelet w low fat cheese	½ cup of oatmeal	Scrambled eggs, one slice of toast
12:00 pm	4oz. grilled chicken, sweet potato	4 oz. Teriyaki salmon/veggies & brown rice	Chicken fajita wraps (grilled)	4 oz. turkey burger with salad.	Chili made with lean ground beef	4 oz. chicken breast, sweet potato	Tofu vegetables stir fry
5:00 pm	Full body	Lower Body	Full Body	Upper Body	Full Body	Yoga	Break
6:30 pm	Protein Shake	Protein shake	Protein shake	Protein shake	Protein shake	Protein Shake	Yogurt/Nuts
7:00 pm	4oz. steak with vegetables	4oz. chicken with asparagus	4 oz. turkey burger with green salad.	4 oz. grilled salmon with green salad.	Stir fry 4 oz. chicken breast with brown rice	Wrap with 4oz. lean ground beef and veggies.	4oz. tuna fish, vegetables

Paleo Diet Example 2

Day	1	2	3	4	5	6	7
Cardio	Break	40 min Cardio	Break	40 minute cardio	Break	40 min cardio	Break
Meal 1	Protein Shake, plus almonds, blueberries	Eggs with vegetables, almonds and raspberries	Protein Shake, plus almonds grapefruit	Eggs with veggies, macadamias, blueberries	Protein Shake and almonds, grapefruit	Eggs with vegetables, almonds, raspberries	Protein Shake, Cashews, Grapefruit
Meal 2	4-6 oz. Chicken salad, tomato, cucumber, onion	4 oz. fish, broccoli, cauliflower	4-6 oz. Asparagus, zucchini	4-6oz fish and mixed green salad	4-6oz. chicken, asparagus, zucchini	4-6 oz. fish, broccoli, cauliflower	4-6oz Chicken salad, tomato, cucumber, onion
Meal 3	½ Avocado	10 raw almonds	½ Avocado	Celery plus one scoop of nut butter	½ Avocado	Celery plus1 scoop nut butter	½ Avocado
Work Out	45 minute cardio	Full Body	45 min cardio	Full Body	45 min Cardio	Full Body	Break
Meal 4	Berries	Protein Shake	Berries	Protein Shake	Berries	Protein Shake	Berries
Meal 5	6 oz. Salmon, mixed veggies	6 oz. chicken & veggie stir fry	6oz. turkey burger, green salad, no bread	6 oz. Steak with roasted vegetables	6oz. chicken, plus vegetable stir fry	6 oz. Chicken burger, no bread, salad	6 oz. Bison, roasted veggies

Meatless (Lacto-ovo Diet)

Day	1	2	3	4	5	6	7
Cardio	Break	40 minute cardio	Break	40 min cardio	Break	40 min cardio	Break
8:00 am	4 egg white omelet with spinach & beans	½ cup oatmeal, 1 scp. protein powder, Almond butter	4 egg white omelet with spinach & beans	½ cup oatmeal, 1 scp. protein powder, Almond butter	½ cup oatmeal, 1 scp. protein powder, Almond butter	4 egg white omelet with spinach and beans	½ cup oatmeal, 1 scp. protein powder, Almond butter t
12:00 pm	1/3 cup of quinoa, Stir Fry with vegetables	Ezekial Wrap/Beans and Vegetables	1/3 cup of quinoa, Stir Fry with vegetables	Ezekial Wrap/Beans and Vegetables	Vegetarian Chili	1/3 cup of Quinoa stir fry with vegetables	Vegetarian Chili
Workout	Full body	Break	Full Body	Break	Full Body	Break	Break
4:00 pm	Black Bean Burger with salad	4 egg white omelet with spinach & beans	1/3 cup of quinoa, Stir Fry with vegetables	4 egg white omelet with vegetables	Ezekial Bread, almond butter, banana, cinnamon	Ezekial Bread, almond butter, banana, cinnamon	Ezekial Bread, almond butter, banana, cinnamon
8:00 pm	Protein shake, 1 tbsp. almond butter	Protein shake, 1 tbsp. almond butter	Protein shake, 1 tbsp. almond butter	Protein shake, 1 tbsp. almond butter	Protein Shake	Protein Shake	Protein Shake

Meal	Nutrition
½ cup oatmeal	83 cal/1.8g fat/14g carbs/**3g protein**
1 cup egg whites	117 cal/0.4g fat/1.8 g carb/**26g protein**
1/3 cup quinoa	160cal/2.5g fat/30g carb/**6g protein**
Ezekiel wrap	150cal/3.5g fat/24g carb/**6g protein**
Vegetarian chili	294 cal/1.2g fat/55g carb/**16.8g protein**
Protein shake (1 scoop)	**15-20g protein**
Black bean burger	294 cal/1.2g fat/55g carb/**16.8g protein**
2 tbsp. Almond butter	195 cal/17g fat/ 6g carb/**8g protein**

Meal Planning & Choices

95% of clients that I work with have no working meal plan. In fact, though many of the "get the idea" of planning a meal, it's rarely done. "It takes too much time." Or "I know what I need in my head." The only question, I have for them is this: "Is it working? Are you winning the battle of the bulge? Are you healthy?" Are you finding a balance in your weekly nutritional intake? The answer is usually, "Not Really."

Meal planning is essential for success. Planning out your meals ensure that you get the right amount of nutrients as well as crowd out any other foods we are trying to move away from. But if it's so effective, why then why don't we all do it? Well, I have generally found that there are two important reasons for us not following through on our meal planning. The first is that it really is not a priority. The second is that we do not really know how to do it.

Let's briefly talk about these two points. The reason that most of us don't plan our meals out during the week is because it really isn't a priority for us. With so many mobile apps, computer software programs, and even your good old pen and paper, we often don't think of it convenient to plan out our weekly meals. In fact, most of us usually just go to the grocery store when we think we need to and randomly pick things up that sound good or look good.

Before we begin a meal plan:

Do you have any food that is not a part of your new healthy habits in your pantry? How about in your cupboards? If you do, it really doesn't make any sense to keep them. If you keep them it will remind you of the way you ate before you started to make change. If you don't think your kitchen or what is in your fridge has any influence on the healthy lifestyle you want to live, think again!

Some Tips on Food Planning:

- **Plan you meals and snacks ahead of time**
- **Get Your fill of Fiber**
- **Canned Foods are often higher in Sodium**
- **Frozen foods are a great option**

Food Substitutions

Replace This	With This
Sugar & artificial Sweetener	Stevia
All Cooking Oils	Organic Cooking Oils
Dairy and Soy Milk	Organic Coconut or Almond Milk
Sports Drinks, Juice, Pop	Water
Chocolate & Candy	Dark Chocolate, Fruit
Grains	Vegetables (high fiber carbs)
Processed, Frozen, Canned Foods	Fresh and Organic (non GMO)
White potato and white rice	Sweet Potato, Brown Rice, and Quinoa
Chips, Granola bars, Sugary Snacks	Nuts/Seeds, Raw Vegetables

Are you too busy to prepare meals?

Whenever I have had very busy times in my life or when I was preparing for a fitness show I was fortunate to have a meal delivery service called Fuel Foods created by my good friend Nick McNaught. The service is great for anyone trying to eat healthy and with a lack of time for preparation. Plus everything on the menu tastes amazing. You go to the website www.fuelfoods.ca and pick your healthy meals for the day that get delivered right to your home. This company is based out of Toronto but I've heard of other companies all over North America.

**Go to
www.totalwellnessbook.com
For FREE tools!**

**Turn this great book into a
wellness support system by
downloading templates,
documents, recipes and other
great tools!**

Chapter 5: Fitness

To lose weight and increase your fitness, you will have to take a look at your fitness plan. In addition, you may have to increase the amount of time and energy focused on exercise. Like other parts of your life, we have to take a look at what you have been doing? You don't want to start running marathons if you don't do so much as walk around your block!

Idea of Problem Spots (belly, love handles, thighs, flabby back

By working out a problem spot (belly, thighs etc.) you are not burning fat in that area. When working out, you do not "spot" reduce fat. You lose body fat in certain places first based on genetics and on your health and hormonal balance.

For example: Thighs being a problem spot usually indicates you have a high amount of chemical estrogens, or Love handles as a problem spot indicates your diet is made up of too many simple carbs. Make sure your thyroid is functional; you get enough sleep, limit stress (not just emotional but physical stress such as poor diet and alcohol)

"Harvard Medical School reports that people who carry significant amounts of belly fat, face a heightened risk for heart disease. The biologically active fat --- medically referred to as visceral fat --- elevates your blood sugar and blood pressure and even lowers your body's amounts of healthy cholesterol. Frequent consumption of alcohol contributes to the elevation of belly fat and threatens your health." (33)

This fat causes metabolic syndrome and chronic inflammation that leads to heart disease and diabetes. Visceral fat literally encrusts the vital organs, the kidneys, liver, stomach, and others. Visceral fat contributes to high blood pressure by squeezing the kidneys, working them and wearing them out. It also drains directly into the liver where it infiltrates, replacing functional tissue with fat. Also causing the "beer belly"

Intensity Workouts:

Certainly Intensity workouts are known to quickly stimulate weight loss faster than other types of workouts. If faster weight loss is wanted, high intense workouts seem to be the best choice. Of course, this is a very high stress body workout and shouldn't be done every day. Your intensity workouts also seem to burn more carbohydrates quickly during the exercise. These work outs last for 10-15 minute intervals of say 1-3 minute reps.

Longer Fat Burning Workouts

Longer fat burning workouts are also great, because they can be done on odd days that you are not doing intense workouts. While they burn off fat during the workout period, they also turn your muscles in to long-term burning fat machines, which is great because it increases your basal metabolism. This means that while pound for pound during workouts, although intense workouts burn more fat, longer fat burning exercise can help you effectively lose weight over the long run.

In both the intensity and long-burn diets our body will start use carbohydrates that you eat before your workout. Therefore I recommend not eating or drinking any sports drinks before working out. If you want to maximize your weight loss, if you want to burn the fastest amount of fat then ideally you want to do so without eating first. So, an early morning workout would be best.

If you're new at this, your first few workouts might be inconsistent. You might quickly fatigue and your muscles might ache – and your body might demand to be fed. But if you do this, you muscles will be better at burning your stores of fat instead of relying on the carbohydrates you just had for breakfast or that sports drink. Long term fat burning workout lasts about 60-90 minutes in -length.

Strength Training/Workouts
Strength or resistance training has obvious benefits. Increases strengths can be helpful for the developing

primed muscles benefits to do a wider variety of exercises.

These exercises are important because:

Unless you are a bodybuilder you should be doing full body workouts. A lot of these exercises are multi joint movements. You want to maximize the workout in the time that you have.

You are going to burn the most calories working more than one muscle. Keeping your rest time minimal and your heart rate up in a HITT style of training (high intensity) you are going to burn fat while increasing muscle for a nice lean toned look... On the other hand if you want to be a body builder this book is not for you ;) As it is not a healthy lifestyle in my opinion.

You can do them from anywhere with free weights or bands. Whether I am training my clients in home with minimal equipment or in a studio gym with all types of machines I always stick to doing resistance training with free weights and your own body weight. There are no excuses this way. No matter where my client is whether at home or traveling they have a bunch of exercise routines they can do from anywhere.

Make sure when using free weights though that your form and technique is perfect! You might want to look into getting a trainer even if it's just for a few sessions to make sure you are doing the exercises properly and you are feeling it in the right place. Or even check out my website for videos. Additionally, ask an experienced friend at the very least. You are not going to get very fit if you are injured. It is better to avoid having that set back. The better your form and knowledge on where you should be feeling each exercise and what you should be focusing on the more you are going to get out of your workout.

Ironically, I hear people tell me all the time that they don't have the energy to exercise; but if you exercise on a regular basis, this actually increases your energy levels. I recommend that they start slowly and gradually over weeks and months build up your exercise tolerance.

Your final goal should be to aerobically walk for 20 minutes per day, 5 days of the week. If fatigue is a problem, then start exercising in small amounts until you slowly build up exercise tolerance, this is especially true for people suffering post viral fatigue syndrome. Low impact aerobic walking built up slowly over a number of weeks isn't a problem but it would be advisable to see your doctor for a health check.

Fine Tuning Your Fitness Routine

Fine tuning would mostly be with form/technique, and being consistent. A fitness routine should be continuously changing as you get in better shape. Otherwise you will plateau.

Burning Fat Tips

To burn fat the bottom line is eating a healthy diet and exercising - getting your heart rate up. To speed up the process drink your share of water and limit chemical exposure. This will ensure other functions of the body are running smoothly. The better you treat your body physically and emotionally the easier it is to be in optimal shape. For example dealing with stress better will lesson cortisol production and you will store less fat in your mid-section.

I know what you're thinking, "Taya, c'mon, this sounds so simple. Will this work?" I feel so confident that if you change your stress levels, eat healthier, keep hydrated, exercise more, and limit yourself from chemical exposure, your weight will tumble, you will have more energy, and you will just feel great. A cornerstone of your new life requires that you address your stress levels.

Cooling Down & Warm Ups

Cooling down and warming is essential to prevent injuries and of course improve our actual performance. Like anything else we do, warming up - or exercising and stretching at slower pace and at a reduced intensity - can help prepare our bodies for aerobic activity and muscle strength training. Cooling down after a good work out helps to reduce our muscle temperature gradually, and reduce to muscle stiffness.

You want to be sure to take the time to warm up. Stretching before any kind of exercise is essential. Far too many people skip warming up and head right to the weights. I have even heard some popular fitness programs give not warming up a green light. Personally, this is a terrible idea. Not warming up can cause injury and increase your "soreness" time. Simply take a few minutes to stretch and warm up.

The purpose of warming up is to get your body to increase its oxygen supply. You can walk, jog or do some light stretches. Consider jumping rope for a few minutes to get going.

The following are some workouts that I recommend that you do for increasing strength, tone, and will help you create the fat burning body that you need!

The Workouts

Workout #1

3/15 jump squats

3/15 squats

3/60 sec wall sit

3/15 Walking lunges

3/15 push ups

3/15 bent over row with bands

3/15 sumo squat + shoulder press (10)

3/15 single leg lunge

3/15 dead lifts

3/15 biceps curl

3/15 shoulder press

Core

3/15 Hanging leg raises

3/25 crunches on ball

workout #2

3/15 jump squats

3/15 walking lunges

3/15 sumo squats

3/15 dead lifts

3/15 bent over row

3/15 reverse fly

3/15 chest press

3/15 fly

3/15 triceps press

3/15 dips

3/15 bicep curls

3/15 shoulder press

3/15 upright row

3/10 plank to push up

3/10 push ups

3/25 crunches on ball

Top Training tips for Body Composition

Experts agree that focusing on muscle building, burning off the fat you do have and getting to the most significant hormone response from exercise are the three essential things to achieving the results we want. Our healthy diet figures prominently in this scenario. Without a doubt what you do to address these areas will have a dramatic effect on your health and your body. After all, you can train all you want, but it will not take you anywhere without proper nutrition.

I have a few training tips for your body composition that I think will help improve the results of your workout:

1. **Increase Your Resting Metabolic Rate (RMR):** This is the rate at which your body burns fat when you are "resting." You can probably see why this is critical since you generally cannot be working out or exercising all the time, right? The level of your RMR is constitutes the majority of the fat that you burn

throughout the day. While working out you certainly burn off energy and fat but when you stretch it out over a week's or months' time it is quite small in comparison.

So how exactly do you increase your RMR? Many experts agree that doing both anaerobic conditioning and strength building are essential because they increase muscle and they burn fat. The focus on anaerobic exercise is that not only does it burn off energy quickly, but it also kick starts your metabolic rate by boosting your level of lean muscle mass. To be sure anaerobic training and strength building will always be essential to fat loss and body composition, so naturally we would want to focus on those two when compared to aerobic training.

2. **Train with high intensity, short breaks:**
   Strength training should be done using high volume exercises and only short rest periods. The more sets you do will speed up the results, but keeping it between 8 – 10 reps in three

sets is a great place to start. Rows, Squats, deadlifts, chin-ups, lunges and bench presses should be the majority of your work out while use weights or resistance in the 75% of your maximum range. Remember this basic rule: Short rest intervals after high powered and intense reps can help burn your fat! In addition, increasing your reps throughout the process is a good way to go.

3. **Train to build muscle:** When you start a program to lose weight, the first thing you want to do is build muscle and stimulate an anabolic response. This is done by burning energy very fast, exercising each muscle group with high intensity. The reason this is so effective is that when the body experience this type of intense workout GH (Growth Hormone) is released into the body in significantly more quantity. GH is a hormone, produced by the pituitary gland that facilitates fat breakdown and boosts the metabolism of glucose and amino acids. GH also has a ripple effect on the body.

Stimulate the release of GH and you also trigger the release of IGF-1 or insulin-like growth factor, which is an essential component of protein synthesis. While you're at it, you'll be releasing the primary anabolic hormone, Testosterone. While Testosterone is released with slightly longer rest periods following very heavy strength and muscle training. What is this tell us? That having a variety of workouts is the best solution! Strength training increases fat burning hormones and burns energy. (34)

4. **The next tip revolves around your priorities** – or what they should be if weight loss and strength gain is what you want. There is no question that performing high intense anaerobic training is essential to burning fat. Regardless of the type of aerobic exercise it's compare to, intense anaerobic training delivers faster and more effective weight loss. The reason for its effectiveness goes back to increase in Testosterone and Growth Hormone which is released.

5. **Maintaining an Active Lifestyle:** Sure you might be going to the gym and eating healthy, but if you're plopping down on the couch every night and living a sedentary life, than you're risking a whole host of problems, the least of which is weight gain. Blood sugar dropping is another problem often associated with a sedentary lifestyle, result in a low metabolism. The best thing to do is continue doing physical activities that you like in between workouts, such as riding your bike, going for a jog or walk, hiking, or playing catch.

More on your metabolic rate

Regardless of exercising, everything you put in your mouth affects the rate of your metabolism, which is the speed that your body burns off calories. Your "basal" metabolic rate is what we want to focus on here because it reflects the amount of calories your body burns while resting. While a variety of factors affect your metabolic rate, your age, gender, and lifestyle's activity level are significant. The "visceral" fat, the fat the lies in our bodies can lead to many chronic diseases. Even if you have temporary positive results from dieting alone, this fat remains. We need to incorporate health and fitness into our lives.

Our bodies are the only "machines" that get better with use. Most other machines or physical objects get worn out, they get dull, and fatigued with more use. But with the right diet, lifestyle, and exercise, your body actually gets better! (35)

Soon you your body will adapt to these positive changes.

By increasing and fine tuning your workouts and eating healthy, your body will begin to come alive. You will start to notice a number of different things including elevated moods, more energy, craving healthier things, greater focus – and of course you will begin seeing your weight drop. But you might also want to be prepared for feeling a bit sore, maybe achy, and even a little tired. Remember that you should start any workout program by first checking in with your doctor. If you are a healthy individual, these feelings will go away. I always view being slightly sore

243

as a sign that my body is healing and getting stronger. You are stretching your body's performance ability and that's okay!

Allow Some Time for Your Body to Rest

I have built some rest times into my plan, but you know your body best. You know when it is important to rest. In fact, consider your "resting" period as "part of" your exercise plan.

Go to
www.totalwellnessbook.com
For FREE tools!

Turn this great book into a wellness support system by downloading templates, documents, recipes and other great tools!

Chapter 6 - Lifestyle/Personal Care Products

Creating a holistic or comprehensive view to health is essential to achieving the health goals we are seeking. This includes taking a deeper look into our overall lifestyle. We can't simply overlook our lifestyle when we are going to make fundamental changes in how we live.

I know that I have already spoken quite a bit on decision making when it comes to the life we lead. Our goals that we have set in place and vision that we hold onto often provide a landscape of how our lifestyle should be.

If you are interested in losing weight and want to clear a distinct path towards wonderful health and fitness, then you will have to try your best to eliminate stress from your life. Abnormal stress for long periods of time can have a negative impact on your body, leading to weight gain, muscle loss, and chronic diseases. The good news is that if you avoid stress and do your best to maintain a mentally and emotional healthy lifestyle, your body will also physically respond in a positive manner.

Effects of Stress on Health

We don't have to a scientist to understand that stress is not good for us. Research has pretty much concluded that repeated exposure to stress in our lives causes havoc on our immune system, depletes our vitamin and mineral levels, and causes everything from colds to heart disease.

Eating healthy, exercising, meditating, and creating an overall healthy lifestyle is essential to combat stress.

Herbal Remedies

Incorporating supplements into your diet can also help you enjoy better health. Here is a short list of some of the supplements that I would recommend to address common ailments.

Valerian – research indicates the valerian improves sleep and the quality of your sleep naturally.

Skullcap – This herb functions as a natural sedative and can be very useful if you have a lot of worry.

Chamomile – Proven to aid in relaxation and promote better quality sleep. Chamomile contains flavonoids, chrysin, and apignein that bind to the nerve receptors which reduces aggression and anxiety.

Kava Kava – This herb jump starts your brain's production of soothing and calming chemicals that help sleeping problems due to anger, anxiety, or fear.

Supplements To Promote Better Sleep

Vitamin B Complex – these family of vitamins are important for the nervous system, which depletes quickly during stressful times. It also helps break down fatty foods, which you may eat during stressful times.

Magnesium - Magnesium has been found to be necessary for nerve function.

Calcium – warm milk anyone? Calcium promotes sleep.

Physical-Mental Activities:

Exercise – We've got this covered but it's worth mentioning again. Increasing your exercise regimen or just getting out for a walk after dinner can help your muscles and your mind.

Warm Showers – A warm sit in a sauna or shower can help relax your muscles.

Prayer – Prayer has been shown to help lower anxiety, reduce fear, and calm the nerves.

Meditation – Like prayer, helping you clear you mind will help you sleep much more sound.

Foods to Avoid if You Want To Sleep Better:
Coffee, chili, tomatoes, potatoes, bacon

The Beauty Product Lie

Sometimes it's hard to hear something negative about group of products that you are familiar with and have used nearly all your life. Chances are that your personal care products are putting you and many millions of people at risk long term damage.

While they smell great and make us feel prettier, we hardly have asked what's inside any of them! What if you were told that many of the chemicals used in our common personal care products can put you and your children at risk for immune problems and may even contribute to some cancers?

Just alongside the growing awareness of food is also a growing awareness of what's inside our personal care products as well.

Consider the following:

- **The contents of eye makeup can be absorbed quickly into our membranes.**

- **Perfumes and hairsprays can irritate our lungs.**

- **Lipstick can be – and usually is – swallowed.**

- **Sunscreen can be absorbed through the skin.**

- **Laundry detergents can irritate our skin and cause allergic reactions.**

Since the average adult in North America uses about nine personal care products every day, means that on average, we are smearing or spraying up to 136 different and unknown chemicals on our body. Some women and some men use up to 15 different chemicals. (36)

A big culprit is sodium lauryl/laureth sulfate, which is one of the most common chemicals in the personal care and cosmetic industry.

Keep in mind that a bit of research has been conducted that has determined that what we put on our skin or inhale can be just as dangerous as the things we actually ingest! Some even suggest that it might even be worse because when we eat something enzymes can actually help break it down and out bodies toxins.

Whereas what we smear on ourselves goes directly into the blood stream entering organs and flushed out only after it has done its damage!

Once these chemicals enter your body, they tend to accumulate over time because you typically avoid the necessary enzymes to break them down. There are literally thousands of chemicals used in personal care products, and the U. S. government does not require any mandatory testing for these products before they are sold.

Many of the same poisons that pollute your environment are also lurking in the jars and bottles that line your bathroom shelves. We all risk becoming a toxic waste dump from the products we use, the foods we eat, and the environment in which we live.

So, what are choices?

Choose Your "Natural" Cosmetics Carefully.

Cosmetics and other beauty treatments are most often applied to the sensitive areas on the face around the eyes and mouth where synthetic ingredients, solvents, mineral oil and other artificial ingredients are most likely to cause a reaction when absorbed into the skin and body.

That's why so many substances in makeup have to be extensively tested before they are considered safe to use—and you may also be surprised to find that some ingredients in major brand cosmetics are still tested on animals.

Why not use something you know is naturally derived? When cosmetics get their color from natural flowers and mineral pigments, it's easier to achieve a subtle, natural look. We feature a selection of foundations, face powders and color cosmetics made with natural pigments to flatter all skin tones and with natural ingredients that provide lasting moisture and rich color.

Sincere there are no federal regulations for beauty products; anyone can claim their product is "natural" or "organic." A label with the word "natural" does not mean the product contains only natural or organic ingredients.

According to the Organic Consumers Association, which has a current "Coming Clean Campaign" aiming to clean up the organic personal care product industry, the word "organic" is not properly regulated with personal care products as it is with food products, unless the product is certified by the USDA National Organic Program.

In fact, some "organic" beauty products contain only a single-digit percentage of organic ingredients. Some brands use ingredients that were simply derived from natural sources but are highly processed and contain synthetic and petrochemical compounds. When it comes to the labeling of cosmetics and body care products, it's kind of a free-for-all. (37)

According to the Environmental Working Group's Skin Deep: Cosmetic Safety Reviews, research studies on SLS have shown links to:

- **Irritation of the skin and eyes**
- **Organ toxicity**
- **Developmental/reproductive toxicity**
- **Neurotoxicity, endocrine disruption, ecotoxicology, and biochemical or cellular changes**
- **Possible mutations and cancer**

If you visit the SLS page on the Environmental Working Group's (EWG) website, you will see a very long list of health concerns and associated research studies. In fact, you will also see their mention of nearly 16,000 studies in the PubMed science library (as well as their link to that list) about the toxicity of this chemical.

There are clearly grounds for concern about using products containing this agent. Yet, skeptics abound who claim that these concerns are overblown and unfounded. It's no wonder that consumers are completely confused about just how much risk this chemical poses.

But high levels of SLS intake, either orally or through the skin, are not ordinarily experienced in normal cosmetics use—**it's the gradual, cumulative effects of long-term, repeated exposures that are the real concern.** And there is a serious lack of long-term studies on ALL of the chemicals in these products— so we don't really know what the long-term effects are.

It's not just repeated exposure to one chemical—it's the combined effect of thousands of little chemical exposures, day in and day out that is of concern. Sorting through the evidence is even more complicated when research findings are exaggerated and misquoted, and then circulated around the Internet as if it were fact.

Real Dangers of SLS—Rumors Aside

A number of studies report SLS being damaging to oral mucosa and skin. This is not at all surprising since SLS is actually used as a skin irritant during studies where medical treatments for skin irritation require an intentionally irritating agent.

A study at the Stern College for Women at Yeshiva University in New York in 1997 examined SLS in mouthwash. They found that SLS in mouth rinses caused desquamation of oral epithelium and a burning sensation in human volunteers. (38)

Links Between SLS, Ethylene Oxide, 1, 4 Dioxane, and Cancer

The evidence linking SLS to cancer is a bit challenging due to the paucity of scientific studies. However, carcinogenic effects are quite possible when you consider that SLS/SLES is often contaminated by two known carcinogens:

1. **Ethylene oxide** (which is what the "E" in SLES represents). A return to the Skin Deep website for ethylene oxide reveals a rating of "high hazard," which appears as an impurity in thousands of personal care products. It is used to "ethoxylate" SLS and other chemicals, to make them less harsh.

2. **1,4 dioxane**, a byproduct of ethylene oxide, also receives a "high hazard" rating from Skin Deep and is associated with an even longer list of common personal care products. On the CDC site, 1,4 dioxane is described as "probably carcinogenic to humans," toxic to the brain and central nervous system, kidneys and liver. It is also a leading groundwater contaminant. I don't know about you, but probably carcinogenic just doesn't sound good enough for me. Avoid it at all costs!

Clean up and green up your daily cleansing and moisturizing regimen.

Skin is your body's largest organ, so you know it has important functions. It is constantly working hard to regulate body temperature, hold in moisture and rid the body of toxins—all the while providing a barrier against infection and the environment. Many soaps, lotions and other skin care products contain artificial and petroleum-based ingredients that may interfere with these functions.

Instead, choose products that don't hinder the skin's natural role of protecting your body. Skin is happiest with a natural regimen of cleansing and moisturizing that features natural oils, botanical extracts and nourishing nutrients. With our cruelty-free, natural products, you get what you need to look good and feel comfortable with your

Many different and "popular" soaps that are found in typical supermarkets and drugstores contain harsh detergents, animal fats, heavy mineral oils, preservatives and artificial colors and fragrances.

How can you get your skin clean by washing it with ingredients like that?

Natural soaps and cleansers are soothing and effective with natural "sudsing" action and cleaning properties. Follow up your cleansing ritual with lotions that contain natural moisturizers, nutrients, antioxidants and pure essential oils. And when selecting a sunscreen, choose from our PABA-free formulas that are water resistant. Natural deodorants are effective because they reduce those bacterial culprits with ingredients such as:

How to Evaluate Your Toxicity

Most people think their exposure to toxins is insignificant. That disease or crazy conditions you read about or hear on television or read online happen to "other" people. The truth is that we are much closer to that story that you might think. While seemingly small amounts of chemical exposure and toxins might not seem like it affects you, there are quite a bit of evidence that is emerging to start thinking that it does.

Take for example, daily use of ordinary, seemingly benign personal care products like shampoo, lotions, toothpaste and shower gels can easily result in exposure to *thousands of chemicals*, and many will make their way into your body and become "stuck" in a bodies, lodge in our fat or organs and tissue. Why do they stay in our bodies? The answer is simple; we simply lack the "natural" mechanisms to break them down.

Over time, this toxic load can become a significant contributing factor to a variety of health problems and serious and chronic diseases, especially if your diet and exercise habits are also not in tip top shape!

Women & Men Versus Chemical Toxicity

Women seem to be predisposed to more autoimmune disorders than men. Diseases such as thyroid disease, fibromyalgia, and multiple sclerosis are far more common in women. Perhaps one of the major contributing factors is that women tend to use far more personal products than men. (37)

Final Tips and Tricks to Lighten Your Toxic Load

Here are a few other suggestions to help you avoid SLS and other nasty chemicals:

• Look for the genuine USDA Organic Seal.

• If you can't pronounce it, you probably don't want to put it on your body. Ask yourself, "Would I eat this?"

• Look for products that are fragrance-free. One artificial fragrance can contain hundreds—even thousands—of chemicals and fragrances are a major cause of allergic reactions.

• Pay attention to the order in which the ingredients are listed. Manufacturers are required to list ingredients in descending order by volume, meaning the first few ingredients are the most prominent. If calendula extract is the last ingredient in a long list, your calendula body wash isn't very natural. (38)

• Stick to the basics. Do you really need 20 products to prepare for your day? Simplify your life.

• Buy products that come in glass bottles rather than plastic, since chemicals can leach out of plastics and into the contents. Bisphenol A (BPA) is a serious concern; make sure any plastic container is BPA free.

• Drink plenty of filtered water every day to assist your body in flushing out toxins.

• Look for products that are made by companies that are earth-friendly, animal-friendly and green. For more information about how to buy cruelty-free, go to Group for the Education of Animal-Related Issues.

BPA Plastic Bottles

Heating plastics or even a fading of plastics in our food and beverage containers emit Zeno-estrogens. Having these enter your system can disturb the health of even the youngest among us. In fact, Zeno-estrogen has been linked to early puberty in females and irregular menstrual cycles. In addition, it has also been linked to causing fatigue, weight gain, loss of sex drive, mood swings, and unstable blood sugar levels, among a whole host of problems.

"BPA" is a synthetic or manufactured estrogen that was first "synthesized" over a century ago. Today it is used in the manufacturing process from such everyday products as plastic water bottles, food containers and baby bottles. (Only recently in 2012 did any legislation get moved to ban the product in everyday products) Since then, laboratory studies have uncovered potential health concerns in a variety of tested animals. (39)

After scientist found that the BPA was horrific, the debate has raged as to what a significant level is. The levels of BPA used in the current experiments were five times lower than that considered harmful for mice, showing that even a low exposure was able to cause noticeable effects in the offspring That's like saying how much poison can we drink until we fall over dead. Shouldn't we just avoid it altogether? Yes, that makes a lot of sense but it doesn't make a lot of profit. You see adding BPA makes the manufacturing process a bit efficient. (40)

Personal Care and Cleaning Products, Brands (Whole Foods, Noah's, Online)

Product + Common Ingredients to avoid	Recommended Brands: +All mentioned brands are biodegradable and not tested on animals
Shampoo/Conditioner/Body Wash Natural Brands – containing no: Parabens Phthalates Sodium Laurel/Laurel Sulfates Synthetic perfumes/Fragrances Petroleum based ingredients Silicones EDTA	1. Shaklee 2. Desert Essence 3. Whole Foods Brand 4. Kiss My Face 5. Burt's Bee's 6. Andalou 7. Alaffia 8. Everyday Shay 9. Dr. Bronner
Toothpaste Natural Toothpastes – containing no: Sodium Laureth/Laurel Sulphates Fluoride	1. Shaklee 2. Toms 3. Comvita
Deodorant Natural Deodorant – Containing no:	1. Shaklee 2. Desert Essence 3. Kiss My Face 4. Hugo Naturals

Aluminum based ingredients Artificial ingredients Artificial fragrances Harsh chemical antiperspirants Preservatives	
Make-Up Mineral make-up Containing no: Bismuth oxychloride Nano & Micro particles Preservatives Unnecessary fillers Talc	1. Faerie Organic 2. Vapour Organic Beauty 3. Real Purity 4. Alima Pure 5. Evan Healy 6. RMS 7. John Masters
Laundry Detergent Natural Detergent – Containing No: Sodium Laureth/Laurel Sophate	1. Shaklee 2. Whole Foods Brand 3. EcoPath

Go to
www.totalwellnessbook.com
For FREE tools!

Turn this great book into a wellness support system by downloading templates, documents, recipes and other great tools!

Chapter 7: Hormones

When we think about our health and fitness, we often forget about the little things that really make a big difference in our lives. Our hormonal system is **one little, BIG thing** that many people forget to talk about when it comes to their health. Today more than ever, our hormonal systems are off balance, causing us to feel fatigued, gain weight, age more quickly, and a number of other negative elements.

Hormonal Imbalance

For women, hormonal imbalance is quite common. In fact, woman between the ages of 25 and 45 can wrestle with hormonal issues.

Though easier to ignore with lighter symptoms the younger you are it may lead to severe conditions as we age. For example, having a hormonal imbalance may lead to depression, anxiety, fatigue, weight gain to urinary infections, uterine fibroids, and endometriosis. (41)

Studies have determined that a hormonal imbalance has its roots in the existing balance in the female body between progesterone and estrogen. A disruption between these two hormones has important consequences in the female's health.

This balance depends on a lot of factors and it can present different aspects from month to month. Factors like stress, diet, exercise and ovulation have an important impact on the hormonal balance in the body. When the amount of one of the female hormones decreases or increases, what happens is hormonal imbalance.

Lack of ovulation is an important factor that can lead to hormonal imbalance. Here is how estrogen and progesterone work in the female body. For 10-12 days from the beginning of a cycle, the body only produces estrogen.

The other hormone, progesterone, is made by the ovaries and this process starts when the ovulation takes place. The level of the two hormones drops only when the menstruation appears. So, if ovulation does not occur, the body has only estrogen and almost no progesterone, and this leads to hormonal imbalance.

Hormonal imbalance can be provoked by a lot of external factors as well. In today's modern world, women lead stressful lives causing them to be exposed to a variety of toxins. Birth control pills, pollution, chemicals used for cleaning in your own home, a poor diet or surgery made on the reproductive apparatus, all can cause an increase of estrogen in the female body. The level of estrogen cannot be balance by progesterone, so hormonal imbalance occurs.

If you think you are suffering from hormonal imbalance, there are some ways to find out if your worries are justified. Some health clinics offer free online tests that you may take if you want to know what is going on inside your body.

How Hormones Effect Your Weight

Our intake of certain foods often influences our balance of our hormones. Today, more than ever we find it easier and easier to buy highly processed, nutrient deficient foods in our grocery stores. Even foods that we consider healthy often don't have the nutritious benefits

Consider the effects of processed soy. Sound healthy, right? Soy is often a meat alternative enjoyed by millions of people. Yet, processed soy contains that "pull down" the thyroid and leads to hypothyroidism.

In addition, soy contains something called phyto-estrogens that often block the absorption of nutrients like Zinc or Magnesium. In fact, processed soy products are often linked to weight gain. As one of the top food allergens that people have, many people get sick and they aren't even sure why! (42)

A Loss of Sleep

Drinking too much caffeine either via coffee, caffeine power drinks, can decrease bone density and stimulate the hypocalmus to generate more cortisol, which is generally produced during stress. This all of course can affect your sleep patterns. (43)

Aspartame, which is common in diet drinks and yogurt, has been linked to destroying the cells in the hypothalamus. The hypothalamus contributes to our body's ability to regulate hunger.

How To Maintain Healthy Hormonal Balance

Certainly among females this maintaining hormonal balance is essential to good health. Imbalances between estrogen and progesterone has been noted to cause many imbalances. (44) For example, a dominance of estrogen often leads to conditions that include water and sodium retention. It has also been noted that during the week prior to menstruation this imbalance has been seen to stimulate carbohydrate cravings. In addition to increases cravings of carbohydrates and other foods, hormonal imbalances have been seen to cause mood disorders, intense PMS, and an increase in fatty weight gain!

All this of course sets off a ripple effect, like a tornado hitting our body's vitamin closet. Vitamin B complex, magnesium, and zinc/copper deficiencies and imbalances in our niacin and potassium levels which all lead to states of depression, mood disorders, water retention! Whew! No wonder it's common to see so many people not feeling good whenever we step out of our house!

Hormones and Proper Diet, and the Impact on our Health

The good news is that our bodies are resilient. Even small alterations can have a dramatic and positive effect on our overall health and the way we feel! Having a well balance diet that provides us with essential amino acids is important and is always a challenge for many vegan and vegetarian diets to satisfy. A healthy and balanced diet that achieves hormonal balance can help us feel more satisfied, help accelerate weight loss, and help us fight off disease.

A diet that consists of fresh fruits and vegetables that provide with nutrient packed and beneficial cellular energy. (45)

Hormone Beneficial Foods:

Berries – Aside from being wonderful to each with just about any meal, berries are packed with antioxidants and fiber.

Broccoli – all with their cruciferous cousins Brussels sprouts, cake, cabbage, and broccoli contains an amazing amount of phytonutrients (isothiocyanates). Basically, these phytonutrients shore up our liver function to help us get rid of toxins that can be devastating to our bodies. They also jump start the production of enzymes that help us rid the body of carcinogens and free radicals.

Flax Seed - containing tons of lignans (phtyoestrogenic compounds) that are known to fight off cancers, including breast and colon cancer. I really love ground Flaxseed because it is so easy for us to add into our cereals, salads, smoothies, and even soups and dressing.

Apples Packed with fiber and antioxidants, consistent consumption of apples can have been shown to reduce osteoporosis, cancer, Type 2 diabetes, and heart disease.

Green Tea - If you are looking for something healthy to substitute your morning coffee, why not try green tea? Just four cups a day and are ready to rock the free-radicals floating around in your system! Green tea extract can lead to increases metabolism, burning fat, and fight off certain cancers – a triple threat to many of the things that are bad in our bodies. Green tea, you might already know, contains polyphenols a powerful antioxidant that reduces inflammation, lowers cholesterol, and helps to balance our sugar.

Red Wine - While I caution about the excess consumption of alcohol, red wine has been noted to have some very helpful effects on the human body.

Here's why: Particular antioxidants found in the seeds of grapes called catechins and resveratrol assist in decreasing inflammation, reducing the risk of heart disease, certain cancers, and help nerve cells. In addition, red wine might be a good after-meal digestive aide. Again, I stress moderation here. Some medical conditions can be aggravated by the consumption of any alcohol, so check with your doctor here!

Virgin Olive Oil - One of my favorite, olive oil has been used for thousands of years and has been noted for having many health benefits when consumed in moderation. Olive oil is rich cancer-busting antioxidants, which are anti-inflammatories. It is also known to aide in controlling high cholesterol. In addition, olive oil has been known to gently reduce our appetite by stimulating the release of a hormone called leptin. What is also great to know is that a diet rich in olive oil has been shown to prevent the accumulation of belly fat. Several studies also show that olive oil helps us to break down deposits of fatty cells!

I heart Avocados - Aside from being a wonderfully tasty treat, Avocado has something called glutathione, which is a very affective antioxidant. Packed with Vitamin E and Potassium, Avocado is a very good for the health of our hearts! Avocado is also filled with a substance known as beta-sitosterol, which has been shown to reduce cholesterol levels.

Yogurt - Probiotics are essential to our health. The good bacteria essentially protect the lining of the colon, help to break down foods, and produces Vitamin K as a result.

Fiber - The truth is we all probably need a little more fiber in our diets. At minimum we need about 35 grams of fiber in our daily diet. Fiber is extremely beneficial because it helps to remove all the excess estrogen that resides in our colon.

Supplements that support our hormones:

Siberian Ginseng, Holy Basil - In his book, The Weight Loss Cure "They" Don't Want You to Know About, Kevin Trudeau, argues that hormones have a huge effect on our bodies, our weight, our health, our metabolism, and how we feel. "The hypothalamus is the body's master gland. It is the master gland that regulates metabolism. It is also the gland that regulates physiological hunger. This glad does not operate in a normal state in fat people. It must be reset to and normalized in order to eliminate intense and constant physical hunger.

The reasons that the hypothalamus is operating abnormally include genetics, a clogged liver, Candida overgrowth, a clogged colon, lack of digestive enzymes, nutritional deficiencies, stress, high fructose corn syrup, artificial sweeteners, microwaved food, MSG, lotions and cosmetics put on the skin, non-prescription and prescription drugs, fluoride and chlorine in the water you drink, bathe, and shower in, dehydration, and lack of water, carbonated drinks, ice-cold drinks, trans-fat, lack of sun, food additives, genetically modified food, heavy metal toxicity, lack of oxygen, environmental conditioning, lack of sleep, EMS, lack of fiber, and several other factors." (46)

Despite our lifelong attack on our hormones the good news is that we can correct it and we can "heal" our system.

Conclusion

A healthy diet isn't a sprint. It doesn't end in 21, 30, or 60 days. Your healthy diet will stay with you for the rest of your life. So think about the daily changes that you can stay with in the long run.

We've covered quite a bit in this book. We focused on goal and vision setting and the importance of maintaining our positive attitude. In addition, we discussed nutrition and the role of our diet in our life style change. While our daily exercise is essential to do, we all need focus on the produces that we buy. These include everyday items such as shampoos, creams, and lotions. These products can impact our hormonal levels and effect how we feel inside and out.

Lastly, I want to encourage you to continue working on your goals every day – even on items that are well beyond the scope of this book.

For more information visit my website at www.tayasfitness.com

**Go to
www.totalwellnessbook.com
For FREE tools!**

**Turn this great book into a
wellness support system by
downloading templates,
documents, recipes and other
great tools!**

About Taya Day

Taya is a personal trainer and fitness model from Toronto. She started competing as a fitness model in 2009 and has won many shows and is a pro competitor with many organizations. Taya has been a personal trainer for over 7 years and trains her clients in-home and out of a private studio in Toronto. (www.tayasfitness.com)

Taya started out as a gymnast and competitive cheerleader, coaching both sports is was what originally got her inspired to be a fitness trainer. She had to learn proper nutrition and fitness (strength, endurance, flexibility) as an athlete to perform her best. She is also inspired and looks up to her grandmother who is a naturopathic nutritionist. Taya has a passion for fitness and health and loves to be a positive role model, and motivate others to complete their goals, to look amazing and to feel amazing.

References:

Eating Free: The Carb-Friendly Way to Lose Inches, Embrace Your Hunger, and Keep Weight Off for Good, Manuel Villacorta, May 14, 2012

Does This Clutter Make My Butt Look Fat?: An Easy Plan for Losing Weight and Living More, Peter Walsh, Free Press; 1, November 11, 2008

The Weight Loss Cure "They" Don't Want You to Know About
Kevin Trudeau, Alliance Publishing Group; Reprint edition March 8, 2011

Webmd.com, 24 July 2012
<http://www.webmd.com/food-recipes/guide/10-tips-for-healthy-grocery-shopping>

GHC.org, 24 July, 2012.
<http://www.ghc.org/healthAndWellness/index.jhtml?item=/common/healthAndWellness/conditions/diabetes/foodBalancing.html>

Mayo Clinic Accessed 24 July 2012
<http://www.mayoclinic.com/health/healthy-diet/NU00200>

Charles Poliquin website. <www.charlespoliquin.com>

WebMed – Food Labeling 24, July 2012
http://www.webmd.com/food-recipes/features/carbohydrates

"Organic/ GMO" by Ronnie Cummins Organic Consumers Association http://articles.mercola.com/sites/articles/archive/2011/10/08/organic-monopoly-and-myth-of-natural-foods.aspx

Charles Poliquin Tip 255: Avoid the Fat Trap: Eat High-Protein, Strength Train, Eliminate Cravings, Supplement

http://www.charlespoliquin.com/Blog/tabid/130/EntryId/881/Tip-255-Avoid-the-Fat-Trap-Eat-High-Protein-Strength-Train-Eliminate-Cravings-and-Supplement.aspx

"Detoxes and Cleanses" by Natalie Jill 24, July 2012 http://nataliejillfitness.com/detoxes-and-cleanses/

"Eat Good Fats" by Charles Poliquin 24 July 2012

http://www.charlespoliquin.com/ArticlesMultimedia/Articles/Article/859/Lose_Weight_for_Summer_Top_Five_Dietary_Tips_For_O.aspx

Accessed September 2012 http://www.livestrong.com/article/128501-negative-health-effects-drinking-coffee/

Accessed September 2012, http://www.huffingtonpost.com/dr-mercola/dairy-free-avoid-this-pop_b_558447.html

"How to Measure Your Metabolic Rate" 24 July 2012 <http://www.dummies.com/how-to/content/how-to-measure-your-metabolic-rate.html>

"On the evils of wheat" Kate Fillion
http://www2.macleans.ca/2011/09/20/on-the-evils-of-wheat-why-it-is-so-addictive-and-how-shunning-it-will-make-you-skinny
www.Mercola.com 24 July 2012

http://www.charlespoliquin.com/ArticlesMultimedia/Articles/Article/859/Lose_Weight_for_Summer_Top_Five_Dietary_Tips_For_O.aspx

1. Eating Free: The Carb-Friendly Way to Lose Inches, Embrace Your Hunger, and Keep Weight Off for Good, Manuel Villacorta
2. Eating Free: The Carb-Friendly Way to Lose Inches, Embrace Your Hunger, and Keep Weight Off for Good, Manuel Villacorta
3. *Does This Clutter Make My Butt Look Fat?,* Peter Walsh
4. *Does This Clutter Make My Butt Look Fat?,* Peter Walsh
5. *Does This Clutter Make My Butt Look Fat?,* Peter Walsh
6. *Does This Clutter Make My Butt Look Fat?,* Peter Walsh
7. Mysuperchargedlife.com
8. Mysuperchargedlife.com
9. http://www.webmd.com/food-recipes/guide/10-tips-for-healthy-grocery-shopping
10. http://www.ghc.org/healthAndWellness/index.jhtml?item=/common/healthAndWellness/conditions/diabetes/foodBalancing.html

11. http://www.mayoclinic.com/health/healthy-diet/NU00200
12. http://www.npr.org/blogs/thesalt/2012/07/16/156854397/some-athletes-reject-high-tech-sports-fuel-in-favor-of-real-food
13. http://www.charlespoliquin.com/ArticlesMultimedia/Articles/Article/859/Lose_Weight_for_Summer_Top_Fi ve_Dietary_Tips_For_O.aspx
14. http://www.livestrong.com/article/128501-negative-health-effects-drinking-coffee/
15. http://www.livestrong.com/article/128501-negative-health-effects-drinking-coffee/
16. http://www.huffingtonpost.com/dr-mercola/dairy-free-avoid-this-pop_b_558447.html
17. "Detoxes and Cleanses" by Natalie Jill
18. "Detoxes and Cleanses" by Natalie Jill
19. http://www.huffingtonpost.com/dr-frank-lipman/sugaraddiction_b_783203.html#s183041&title=Have_A_Piece
20. Manuel Villacorta
21. Manuel Villacorta
22. GHC.org, 24 July, 2012. <http://www.ghc.org/healthAndWellness/index.jhtml?item=/common/healthAndWellness/conditions/diabetes/foodBalancing.html>
23. Paleo Diet.com
24. Paleo Diet.com
25. http://www.webmd.com/food-recipes/features/carbohydrates
26. The Weight loss Cure, *"They" Don't Want You To Know About*,
27. *New England Journal of Medicine* sheds a bit of light the long term physiological influences of severe calorie restriction

28. http://www.webmd.com/food-recipes/features/carbohydrates
29. Kevin Trudeau
30. Charles Poliquin.com
31. http://wheyoflife.org/health-benefits/wellness-whey-protein/
32. Charles Poliquin.com
33. Charles Poliquin.com
34. http://www.dummies.com/how-to/content/how-to-measure-your-metabolic-rate.html
35. "Detoxes and Cleanses" by Natalie Jill 24, July 2012 http://nataliejillfitness.com/detoxes-and-cleanses/
36. Organic Consumers Association Organic/ GMO
37. Organic Consumers Association Organic/ GMO
38. Chemical Toxicity
39. http://www.dukehealth.org/health_library/news/10086
40. http://www.dukehealth.org/health_library/news/10086
41. Hormonal Imbalance - Kevin Trudeau
42. Hormonal Imbalance - Kevin Trudeau
43. Hormonal Imbalance - Kevin Trudeau
44. Hormonal Imbalance - Kevin Trudeau
45. Hormonal Imbalance - Kevin Trudeau
46. Hormonal Imbalance - Kevin Trudeau

For more updates, fitness articles, and videos, please visit:

www.tayasfitness.com

**And...Go to
www.totalwellnessbook.com
For FREE tools!**

**Turn this great book into a
wellness support system by
downloading templates,
documents, recipes and other
great tools!**

www.ingramcontent.com/pod-product-compliance
Lightning Source LLC
Chambersburg PA
CBHW060837280326
41934CB00007B/824